Gameful Healing

Almost a Memoir;
Not Quite a Parable

Book 2

in Series

"Gameful Life"

Victoria Ichizli-Bartels

Gameful Healing
Almost a Memoir; Not Quite a Parable
Book 2 in Series "Gameful Life"
1st Edition

Copyright © 2020 Victoria Ichizli-Bartels

The moral right of the author has been asserted.

All rights reserved.

Cover design by Alice Jago

All trademarks and brands mentioned in this book are for clarifying and reference purposes only. Rather than putting a trademark symbol after every occurrence of a trademarked name, the names are used in an editorial fashion and to the benefit of the trademark owner, with no intention of infringement of the trademark. Where such designations appear in this book, and where the author (and publisher) was aware of that claim, they have been capitalized. The trademarks and brands are proprietary to their owners and are not affiliated with this document in any way.

The sources to the quotations made in the book are given before, after, or in the same places as the quotes in the text.

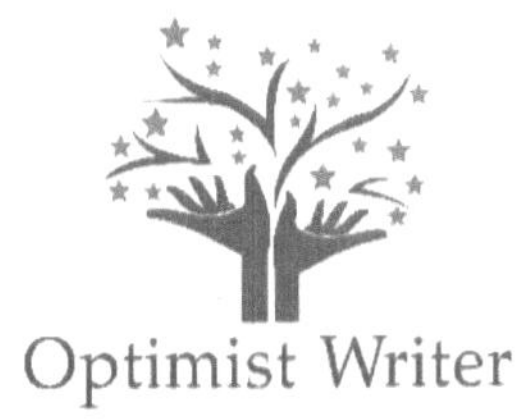

Optimist Writer

*"Some things in life are out of your control.
You can make it a party or a tragedy."*

— Nora Roberts,
Vision in White
("Bride Quartet")

Table of Contents

Table of Contents 8

Gameful Life Series and Self-Gamification 10

1. Introduction 13

2. Chronology 23

3. Learning...27

4. Parable 31

5. Memoir 41

6. Anthropology 48

7. Kaizen 54

8. Gamification...59

9. Self-Gamification..64

10. Healing...68

11. My Body 75

12. Food Intolerance..81

13. The Dentist 84

14. The Doctors 87

15. An Alternative 94

16. The Symptoms 98

17. Nutrition Plan...102

18. Weight...106

19. Gameful Life 110

20. Fun......117

21. Gluten, the Mine......123

22. Ataxia or Not 132

23. Milk, the Creeper......145

24. Carbohydrate-Protein-Thalassemia Puzzle......150

25. Going Nuts (and Seeds) 161

26. Sorbitol Bug......164

27. Eyes and Foggy Vision 169

28. Perfume......177

29. Arthritic "Rubik's Twist" 184

30. The Daily Games 196

31. Now It's Your Turn 209

Further Reading......215

Acknowledgments 221

About the Author 224

By Victoria Ichizli-Bartels......226

Gameful Life Series and Self-Gamification

The resources listed here are those available at the time of publishing. For the full list of available resources on Self-Gamification, which grows continually, go to www.victoriaichizlibartels.com/self-gamification/

Book Series "Gameful Life" addresses various aspects of Self-Gamification separately. Check out the books available so far in this series:

Gameful Project Management is a Self-Gamification Based Awareness Booster for Your Project Management Success (Gameful Life Book 1): www.victoriaichizlibartels.com/gameful-project-management/

This book, *Gameful Healing*, is Book 2 in the series: www.victoriaichizlibartels.com/gameful-healing/

More books in this series are in progress. Find out on the Self-Gamification page (the link at the top of the page), which these are.

Stand-alone books:

Self-Gamification Happiness Formula addresses Self-Gamification in detail. You can check it out here: www.victoriaichizlibartels.com/self-gamification-book/

5 Minute Perseverance Game is a short, fun book, which I wrote before I had heard about gamification and kaizen, two of the three approaches Self-Gamification brings together. I invite you to check it out here: www.victoriaichizlibartels.com/5-minute-perseverance-game/

Online course

Motivate Yourself by Turning Your Life Into Fun Games is an online course on Udemy with a couple of hours of content on Self-Gamification, a unique self-help approach uniting anthropology, kaizen, and gamification. www.udemy.com/course/motivate-yourself-by-turning-your-life-into-fun-games/

Self-Gamification community

To find out how you can join, visit this link: www.victoriaichizlibartels.com/community/

1. Introduction

I never wanted to have health issues. But I have. For most of my life.

I never wanted to be different. Or at least not *too* different. Yes, I wanted to be unique to my family and friends. But in general, I tried to fit in, and be like everyone else. And, at first sight, it might seem like I was.

But after a second glance it would become apparent that I wasn't. I was sure that people thought I was just being picky about my food (I imagined them thinking: *Is she a fitness freak?*); I couldn't see properly but didn't wear either glasses or contact lenses (*Picky about that too?*) since I got migraines from wearing glasses (*Really?*); I frequently had a runny nose (*She must have some kind of virus!*); and never participated in sports (My thoughts: *I wish I could! Why am I not able to?*). I hated it when people started looking at me as if they liked me, talking to me, or spending time with me, but then were dumbfounded when these strange tendencies became apparent, and I felt I needed to explain them.

Today there is a term for such unseen differences between us. It is "neurodiversity," which "refers to variation in the human brain regarding sociability, learning, attention, mood and other mental functions in a non-pathological sense." – Wikipedia[1]. Today, many great activists are working toward including everyone in our societies, whatever challenges or conditions they might face. One such activist is Will Wheeler, who has many followers on LinkedIn and his website TheDyslexicEvolution.com[2], using the brilliant tagline "Embracing Difference".

But that is today. In the years between the start of this story and the very recent past, such a term either didn't exist or wasn't widely known.

So, if I was supposedly different, then why wasn't it visibly? That would've been easier, right? Then people would avoid me at first glance, rather than doing so only after getting to know me, and then with disgust (as I thought) or strange looks, which I interpreted as them thinking me persnickety. Getting judged at first glance would be better than on the second, right? Now I realize how deluded such a belief was, but back then I could only see and feel my discomfort at being the way I was.

I guess my story of being different began long ago, with my predecessors and those things I inherited, but my particular medical conditions started as a toddler. I got very sick then, which moved a doctor to suspect rickets and prescribe treatment with radiation. Later, in school, I fainted more than once, and after some tests and blood analysis, I was diagnosed with anemia. My mom made it

---

[1] https://en.wikipedia.org/wiki/Neurodiversity
[2] https://www.thedyslexicevolution.com/

possible for me to go on summer vacation to a sanatorium. There, at least once, I had to stay in bed due to low body temperature, while everyone else went to the beach.

Then, in my late twenties, I got Bell's palsy on my right side, and doctors couldn't say why. Recently, my eye-doctor and optician discovered that Bell's palsy might have been responsible for my current eye condition, which doesn't permit me to wear either glasses or contact lenses for my short-sightedness. Until then I'd thought the only effect of the Bell's palsy was to cause the corners of my mouth to move differently when I smiled. But it seems it also affected my eye movement. The muscles on the right seem to be considerably slower than those on the left.

My latest adventure is osteoarthritis. I became aware of it thanks to an aching left shoulder. It started with something just being off whenever I moved my arm forward, like a bit of wood peeled off a door and scratching on the frame, but then it developed into a sharp pain. That pain made me aware of the pain in other joints too. I had experienced a burning sensation in my knees before, but simply ignored it. I sit and walk with a slightly bent back due to lower back pain, but I always thought I was just too lazy to maintain better posture. The joint on my right wrist hurt for quite a while, and I can't hold anything in my right hand for too long, especially if it is heavy. But I thought it was just repetitive strain from crafting. It surely wasn't a chronic condition requiring painkillers. I had vowed not to take medicine anymore. Well, OK, OK, I was fine with food supplements, but painkillers?!

And then, I talked to my mom, and complained to her about my joint-ache discovery. I knew she had problems with her joints too, but what she told me was a shock. "I've had it since before you were born. I remember the doctors trying all kinds of treatments, with salts and heating, but nothing helped. You learn to live with it."

I Googled arthritis, and it can certainly be hereditary.

But this pain sucks! I now understand why I gradually stopped doing my beloved workout and yoga, which I practiced for over half a year and enjoyed enormously. All that joint ache stopped enticing me to get down on the floor and do the exercises.

My mom is very mobile in her eighties, so she's living proof that you can live with arthritis — and in her case quite a few other conditions — comparatively well. But to experience pain so often? I didn't want to. I tried really hard to be pain-free and normal. Others were normal, but not me. Why?

But it looked like I was in a vicious circle.

As soon as I thought I had got one thing under control, another strange thing appeared. There always seemed to be something about me that was different from other people. Until recently, I hated the need to explain these differences with all my heart.

Besides wishing I had the full range of movement in my eyes and my entire body, I also always wanted to be able to eat anything I wanted. But I couldn't. I now realize this has been the case for most of my life, but most acutely in the last third.

For a long time I thought my stomach aches could only be cured with medicine. Wasn't there a pill for everything? Apparently not.

For me, dieting was only about weight-loss, not for use in regaining health and well-being, or to reduce pain.

Just before my husband and I moved from Germany to Denmark in 2008, a doctor suggested I try a specific and entirely new nutrition plan. He sent me to one of the local healthy grocery stores, where I could buy gluten and lactose-free bread. It was an out-of-this-world experience.

I still remember how the shop looked inside, or rather how the shelves with various kinds of gluten-free bread looked, and how the light flooded the interior through the windows. I also remember not knowing what to choose: corn, buckwheat, millet, or rice bread? They all looked so different from what I was used to. If I remember correctly, I bought several — some made from just one gluten-free flour, others from a mixture — so that I could taste them all. Despite having eaten buckwheat as a child, knowing what rice tasted like, and enjoying Mamaliga, a traditional Moldovan and Romanian polenta dish made of cornflour, I still couldn't fathom that there was bread made out of all these. And millet was so far removed from my world that I couldn't think of it at all.

The experience of eating differently was even more amazing when the pain almost magically receded, without the need for antacids or other stomach medicine. I also began losing the extra weight I had gained in the previous decade, without even trying.

Over ten years have passed since then. I have learned a lot; I've read many books and articles, joined celiac communities in Germany and Denmark, and started explaining food intolerances and sensitivities to others.

Over those ten plus years, people told me again and again, "You seem to know so much; you know, you could write a book about your experiences. It could help other people in a similar situation."

But I resisted, because I thought I didn't want to write about such a heavy topic. Today, as I approach my whole life gamefully, I am aware that my health situation was hard because I resented it instead of wholeheartedly embracing it as a part of me.

I don't know how long this resistance might have continued. But I know that at the end of 2018, things changed, and quite drastically.

First, I had the idea to write fiction that incorporated challenging health conditions. I was intrigued and started planning, first a romantic short story, and later a whole novel.

Then I started reading modern parables about how to have success in business and life, as well as how to become financially independent. I loved the idea of writing fiction that featured true feelings and experiences, and that taught life lessons.

At the same time, I realized for whom I wanted to write such a book in the first place: my children, Niklas and Emma. If they ever have to face similar challenges — and I've learned that food intolerances can "erupt" in a person's thirties or forties (they did for me; I am forty-seven at the time of writing) — then I want them to have access to my experiences, so they have something to relate to and can feel supported as they navigate such health issues.

After several failed attempts to write the first chapters of the parable — in which I tried to squeeze in my whole story so far — I became aware that what I needed to write was a memoir. A memoir could take any shape and be whatever length I liked, allowing me to share my adventure and what I had learned through it.

However, the style of a parable offered the brilliant possibility to summarize lessons learned into a story.

On top of all that, I currently can't stop reading many books in parallel, combining fiction with non-fiction.

And since what is fun for us is the best compass, then that is what this book is: a memoir featuring a parable. Although the style is a mixture of two genres, it is basically about how to navigate health surely, securely, and with a light, kind, gameful, and simultaneously honest and courageous attitude.

Here is another inspiring influence on the shape this book seems to be taking. My children, my husband, and I enjoy reading together *Good Night Stories for Rebel Girls* by Francesca Cavallo and Elena Favilli, and *Stories for Boys Who Dare To Be Different* by Ben Brooks. These books tell you about the whole lives of inspiring people in short, gripping stories. Thus, I made each of the chapters in this book as short and stand-alone as possible. It was fun to turn each element into a piece that a reader could easily cover in a cozy fifteen-minute coffee break, or in some cases a much shorter one.

I recommend that you read this book as if it was a novel, from beginning to end, without taking notes, and without taking anything too personally.

Remember that I am not a medical doctor, and I don't make any suggestions about how you could or should act in your situation. This is my personal story, which continues to evolve from one day to another. You could say I am my own case study, as you are yours.

Since this book deals with the medical conditions I contend with, I mention the doctors and other medical personnel and health specialists that help me. I don't use their names here, and have done so deliberately to protect their identities. I don't want the possible misinterpretation of my interactions with them to harm or affect them in any way. All of the doctors I've encountered were eager to help, and did the best they could. If their advice didn't bear fruit at any point, it was primarily due to my resistance to listen to what they had to say from their point of view, or some misunderstanding on my part (which is the same thing). I can only recall one doctor, many years ago, who was eager to deceive me for profit, and they are not featured in this book; I only vaguely remember our encounter.

I have had many wonderful physicians over the years, mainly because we moved a lot, either within one city, between different cities, or even between countries. In some cases, the text might read as if I mean the same physician, when in fact this was two or more different persons. I might make reference to my physician as him or her, depending on who it was at that specific time. I don't differentiate more fully between different doctors because the story doesn't require it.

I hope you enjoy this journey with me. I hope this book adds value to your life, but that it does so imperceptibly, without making you feel uncomfortable. I hope it will inspire you to look kindly, lightly, honestly and non-judgmentally at your life's adventure, be it in navigating the sea of your mind and body's responses to various triggers, or something else, as I continue learning to do every day.

2. Chronology

I hope that the purpose of this book is straightforward. As you might have seen in the dedication, I wrote this book primarily for my children. If they ever experience even remotely similar challenges to me, I want them to have examples of how to live with and make the best of them. They already have experience with a challenge that is invisible to others at first. Both have asthma and need various medical products to bring their breathing back to normal. I get inspired by them every day, and we learn together how to master such hidden challenges. We support each other in the process.

Like any parent, I have a big wish for my children. I wish for them to recognize that any challenge they face can be seen like a game whereby they can "level up" in almost any situation. And I hope that they, and you (if you are not one of my children), can get some inspiration from the bundle of stories I tell in this book.

But how should I tell my story? As this is a memoir, I have consulted the many memoirs I have read or am reading now (I always read several books in parallel. I probably should count how many memoirs are in there... As far as I can see from my desk when I turn around, there are at least five memoirs and a couple of biographies on the bookshelf containing the books I'm currently reading, not including the ones on my Kindle).

Some memoirs are written chronologically, others are not.

There is no particular sequence here: just a current bubbly thought containing scraps of memories, pouring out onto the page.

Also, I can't guarantee that my memories are accurate. At first, I was horrified by this realization. But then tremendously relieved when I found the following quote by Rachael Herron, who wrote, in her utterly helpful book for memoir writers *Fast-Draft Your Memoir*, "Our memories are changing all the time."

Herron quotes Daniela Schiller at Mount Sinai Medicine, who "showed in a landmark study in Nature (2010) that memories transform every time they're recalled," to have said the following, "Every memory is fabricated, and the past is nothing more than our last retelling of it."

So all I can do is tell you what I remember today. I researched as much as possible, but in some cases all I had were these scraps of memories. However, it was fun to explore, and to discover that, in some cases, I put the puzzle pieces in the wrong places. So no chance of chronology, but I have attempted to create some structure for you to follow.

In any case, you are in for a wild ride!

I don't mean because my thoughts and memories are strange or bewildering, although they sometimes are (as well as hilarious, if I don't take them too seriously or personally, which is not always easy).

But because I intend to have fun in the process. I have preached the following for several years now: "Have your Fun Detecting Antenna on." This extraordinary device is nothing else but an awareness of what is fun for you, and ensuring it is always detecting fun, whatever you are up to.

Imagine that you are doing something and enjoying it, but then at some point you observe yourself no longer having fun. With your Fun Detecting Antenna on, you would stop what you are doing, notice any complaints you have, or if you are upset or angry (i.e. become aware of what is happening inside and outside of you, non-judgmentally), and then detect whatever move from where you are that would be fun. Or maybe you add a fun element to what you are doing, and with that, make the direction you are moving in fun. But the key is to stop and become aware when something stops being fun, and then boldly address it.

I must admit that I used to, and still sometimes do, forget about this, and instead have the "I have to conform to my idea of the stereotype of others" device on.

But thanks to my joints and constant confrontation with pain and discomfort, and the reminder that I won't always be here, and who knows for how long, I want to have fun. An enormous amount of fun. Including right now, as I write these words. And I do. So that is the right way to go. Because "if we are not having fun, we are moving in the wrong direction." – Ariel and Shya Kane

I still want to explore all the adventures I've had with various health challenges, and in doing so help others, but I also want to have fun in the process. And in that way, as I have learned, I will serve you, the reader, in the best possible way.

That is because only if I manage to design and play my life in a fun and happy way, with all its bumps of health adventures, can I convey this possibility to you.

I tell my children often that my biggest wish for them, their father, members of our family, our friends, and myself, in addition to the one above, is that we all live long, happy, and healthy lives. And for these three wishes to come true and unfold together.

Dear reader, if you haven't found yourself listed in the paragraph above, then please feel included in all the good wishes of this chapter, and the whole book.

But let's remember that happiness includes having fun.

I wish us all fun, every step of the way. So double-check that your Fun Detecting Antenna is on, and if it points toward reading this book further, then turn the page and read on.

3. Learning

There is no fun without adventure. And "Fun is another word for learning." — Raph Koster, *Theory of Fun for Game Design*

And so I learned, and I am still learning, during my undertaking of writing this book, and exploring my adventures with my health.

That is my very personal adventure and learning curve.

You are having your own in your life.

But, as a gamer (whether you are one already, or you are in the process of becoming the gamer in your life by becoming aware of the possibility), you will know that looking over the shoulders of other gamers, to see how they play their games, can give you ideas and inspiration on how to manage the same levels.

So, I hope that "looking over my shoulder" will help you in navigating your own gameful life and health.

You might — as many do — enjoy watching YouTube to find out how others play your favorite games. My children love that, and children today often say that they want to become YouTubers when they grow up.

For me, I like to "watch" and learn by reading books.

I also learn from members of my family, friends, doctors, other medical personnel, and health specialists, who give me advice on various ways to take care of myself.

But here are a few more words on the book-teachers I learned from, both before and during the writing of this book. I will continue learning from these and other books, by reading some for the first time, and re-reading others.

Since this book is mostly a memoir, I read and looked into books about the craft of writing memoirs, as well as reading or re-reading inspiring memoirs by many great, and hilarious, people.

For the parable part (and I am still going to write parables within the "Gameful Life" series, even if this book isn't one), I continue to discover books that offer advice and life lessons.

To continue being inspired as a writer, I consult many books on the craft of writing (in addition to the one specifically on memoirs) and how to be a professional writer, whatever the circumstances. This includes the topics of maintaining a healthy lifestyle as a writer, as well as how to be a writer while living with chronic illnesses.

To sharpen my skills in awareness and living in the moment, I continue to read the amazing books by the award-winning authors, and my dear friends, Ariel and Shya Kane.

When I wish to recall how to do all of that in small steps, and to bypass my fears, I call on the books by Robert Maurer. I will tell you more about him later in this book, in the chapter about kaizen.

I also learn from those who embrace pain instead of resisting and fighting it, cope with challenges invisible to others, turn their health challenges into games, and find the strength and confidence for everyday courage.

I am learning how to be kind, honest, and helpful to myself and apply gentle pain relief techniques. And how to fuel my body in the best possible way.

In this book, I will quote these authors and their books several times. You can also find the books I learned and am still learning from in "Further Reading."

I am also reading many other books in parallel or succession to these. Books are my favorite teachers. They are always there for me, whatever the time of day, and are in no hurry to be read. As in the many areas where I want to learn more, I chose them to guide me while I practice navigating the sometimes stormy, sometimes quiet sea of intolerances, pain, and other challenges.

I was excited but also scared to embark on this adventure of going back into my memories, as well as exploring the present and becoming more aware of my bodily responses and my thought processes.

So, let's see what happened.

4. Parable

Let me tell you about that parable.

It all started with a writing competition.

Well, there is, of course, a backstory to it. But first, here is how the adventure of the book you are reading now started.

At the end of 2018, I discovered a Christmas short story contest on Goodreads, organized by Support for Indie Authors[3]. Almost immediately a story came to mind, complete with ideas for its structure and a title: *You Are What You Don't Eat.*

The story was of a young woman, Viviana, or Vivi for short, with a severe gluten sensitivity. She was reluctant to talk about it, often disguising her refusal to eat anything from a bakery with a wish to stay healthy. She would rather be snickered at for being a fitness freak than pitied for being sick or "abnormal."

She joined an event at a pizzeria with an open oven. This restaurant was one of those enticing places where they

---

[3] https://www.supportindieauthors.org/short-story-contest

prepare meals – including pizzas – in front of their patrons.

Right from the moment Vivi saw the oven in the center of the restaurant, Vivi knew coming here was a bad idea.

She chose a seat as far from the kitchen area as their reserved table would allow, ordered antipasti, and hoped for the best.

But after some time, the flour in the air entered her mouth. Vivi could feel its powdery texture. In response, her body sent violent signals of protest.

Her stomach tripled in size; as a result her chest was squeezed by her bra and Vivi could hardly breathe.

After failed attempts to brush off her symptoms and try to enjoy the evening, Vivi gave up. She mumbled excuses to her company, paid hastily, and ran out of the restaurant. She stopped on the corner outside to catch her breath and replace the floury air of the pizzeria with the fresh, cool December air.

The pizzeria owner's handsome son followed after her, demanding to know what the matter was and whether he could help.

At first, Vivi shook her head, but after some pressing questions from Luca, the handsome Italian, Vivi reluctantly shared her gluten issues with him.

It was intended that Luca would inherit his mother's pizzeria. He wasn't keen on the idea, but he did love helping there. He was wondering what he could do with his life. He knew it would be in gastronomy, but he wanted something different from his mother's pizzeria or his brother's espresso cafe.

Meeting Vivi distracted Luca from his normal routine.

After she ran out of the restaurant and he caught up with her, Luca insisted on bringing Vivi home and waiting while she took a shower, changed into something clean and put her clothes contaminated with wheat flour on to wash.

Then they talked.

I wasn't sure at that time whether Luca and Vivi knew each other before this incident.

I am still not, since I am no longer pursuing this storyline. This book here happened to take on a completely different shape, format, and even genre. I might never find out. Maybe someone else will find out. Or maybe I will write the story of Vivi and Luca in a completely different way. Who knows. All I know right now is the beginning (or middle, depending on when in the story the scene above takes place) and the end, which I will uncover later in this book — no spoilers for now.

Instead, let's go back to the true story about creating the fictional one about Vivi. So, about a month before

Christmas 2018, I set out to write a short story about someone suffering from gluten and possibly other food intolerances.

The inspiration for this creative impulse was something I witnessed at a local writers' club meeting.

At this meeting, a new member made an intriguing suggestion to one of our hosts. Our host has struggled with several chronic illnesses for many years, and this new member asked if she had ever thought of using these experiences as a feature for a protagonist or other character in her novels. Our new member had read a crime novel where the author drew on his wife's illness. Our host was pensive. She said she would have enough material, since she had researched her rare combination of genetic diseases, and participated in internet forums to learn and share experiences with others. She shared that she, in fact, had already started such a story, featuring a character with a rare genetic disease.

While I listened to them, I asked myself whether I would write about my food sensitivities. The answer was "No" again. I say "again" since, as mentioned in the introduction, many people upon learning of my food intolerances have suggested I write a self-help or other book about it. But my answer was always "No" because I resented being sensitive to so many types of food. I didn't want to write about something bad and depressing, did I? Of course not! And being intolerant to food was depressing. Or so I thought.

But the idea of writing a fictional story had been planted in my head, and the writing contest sent this into action. I started plotting and writing the story. I had immense fun and it soon became clear that it would not fit into a short story. I also prefer to read novels or novellas, over short stories. I occasionally observe myself worrying that if it takes me less than fifty minutes to read a non-fiction book then it won't contain all the necessary material I am interested in, hence I love the books I read to be medium length: not too long and not too short.

So it looked like I had a novel in development. I considered what I enjoyed reading, and although I had never written a romance before, I decided to give it a try. The presence of two characters, Vivi and Luca, made this a logical choice. And my love for Nora Roberts' books, with her ability to mix various genres with that of a romance, whilst simultaneously tackling serious issues, inspired me to go in that direction. I set about developing the plot.

As much as outlining the book progressed, the writing of it stalled. I didn't seem to have any wish to write it. Instead, I wrote other books — non-fiction ones.

Maybe I didn't want to replicate my idol's work. Even if Nora Roberts has never – to my knowledge – written about food sensitivities, it still felt like coloring in someone else's design in a coloring book, rather than creating my own painting. It seemed I wanted to set my own pattern, but I didn't know how.

Around that time, I discovered another genre — the parable.

I had read a few parables in my life. *Who Moved My Cheese?* by Spencer Johnson was the most recent, following those read at school and long since forgotten.

I rediscovered this genre not that long ago. I previously published a book for writers called *Cheerleading for Writers*, and was curious to find out what the writers who read and reviewed my book were writing. I was thrilled to discover that successful and acclaimed authors valued my book, and that I could also read and enjoy their brilliant works, which I otherwise might not have discovered. One of the reviewers was a New York Times bestselling author John David Mann. The Go-Giver books, which he co-authored with Bob Burg, sounded very intriguing, and I ended up reading all of them, as well as the other parables he co-wrote with other authors.

I was inspired and thought, "I also want to create something like that."

That was how I replaced the charming Luca with a young woman to be Vivi's inspiring mentor.

I quickly had a name for the mentor. My friend Jennifer Nekuda, Jen, started a blog entitled "Gone With The Weight"[4] with the tag-line "One woman's journey of

---

[4] https://gonewiththeweightblog.com/

food, fitness, and fun." As soon as I had the idea for the parable, I knew I wanted her to be Vivi's mentor. The reason was simple. In many of her posts Jen had "mentored" me, without even intending to. Although she was on a quest to reach a healthy weight through diet and exercise, I, being slightly underweight, was looking for something different.

I was looking for more foods I could eat without getting a stomach ache. Still, her epiphanies helped me along the way. Most memorable was the question in one of her blog posts: "The body can talk to you... are you listening?"[5] She wrote that we need to eat to fuel our bodies, but many of us eat when we either don't need additional fuel, or we need a different kind of fuel to what we consume. The conclusion to this blog post was highly enlightening and encouraging,

"In present time, I eat when I'm hungry. In doing so, I find I don't overeat. And I find when I do eat, I eat until I'm satiated and satisfied. I have surprised myself by how little food is needed to do the activities I want to do. I have quit eating just because something tastes good. I have learned what my body wants for fuel, and by listening and paying attention to what my body is saying, I have a choice. I look, and I listen and let my body tell me what it wants, and I do what it tells me. I don't listen to the brat in my thoughts anymore who

---

[5] https://gonewiththeweightblog.com/2018/10/05/the-body-can-talk-to-you-are-you-listening/

says, like a child throwing a temper tantrum – 'I want it NOW!'" – Jennifer Nekuda

While reading this post, I recalled how I used to misinterpret the pain in my stomach with a pang of hunger. But in truth, it was just a helpless cry for me to stop eating what was not good for me. As soon as I found a diet that was gentle on my stomach and my body, I started to recognize when I was satisfied, and no longer over-ate.

After fretting over it for a few hours, I found the courage to ask Jen if I could feature her as the mentor for the main character in my parable. She was excited about the idea, and offered to help where she could.

I again started enthusiastically outlining the story, and making notes on scenes.

But there was another surprise on the way. Vivi's story stopped being concise and about only one challenge. I based her character on my life, but I didn't want her to be completely me. So there was a conflict.

If I wanted to share my challenges and experiences with my children, Vivi had to be more rather than less like me. I put this worry aside for some time, relying on discovering the answer later, and set off to write the first scenes of the book. After writing several irrelevant scenes and "dancing around" (which was procrastination), I neared the scene where Vivi meets Jen. Eager to emulate the conflict in the fiction books I loved, I made Vivi resent Jen for being one of her sister's best friends. And to show Vivi's discomfort with food, I had her helping prepare the food for her little sister Ana's thirtieth birthday.

So, I wrote and rewrote this scene, reluctant to address the dialogue of Vivi and Jen's first encounter. I had just some brief excerpts of their interaction and a general description of the scene.

Then, after working on it some more, I decided to read some of it to the members of my local writers' club. Previously I had shared parts of the romantic novel I initially outlined, and they liked it. So I was hoping they would also appreciate this new plan for a parable.

I was wrong. Ever-so subtly and kindly, whilst trying not to hurt my feelings and expressing how much they value my opinion and respect me as an author, all those who shared their opinion said in one way or another, "That's not what I would read." Which, upon reflection, meant that none of them liked it.

On the bus home after the meeting, I could see it too. It was bad, really bad. The frequent use of the word "cheese" was just one sign. There were, in fact, four occurrences of this word in the thousand-word excerpt. In a subsequent meeting we laughed together about all that cheese, and I thanked my fellow writers for their frankness.

Their honesty helped me to be honest with myself, and to realize that neither parable nor fiction alone was the best vehicle for me to tell my story.

Something else was, which I'd felt drawn to for some time but had resisted for many years — despite secretly downloading and reading many articles on the writing of. A memoir.

5. Memoir

Yes, in a memoir, I would be able to tell my story as it was, and my children wouldn't have to guess what in Vivi's story was mine and what was not.

They would want to know how I mastered what I had to master, because together with my husband, I am the closest to them genetically, and hopefully also spiritually.

Yes, they would probably be more interested in my adventures than anyone else.

I don't exactly know why I resisted writing a memoir so much in the past. Although the wish was always there, one of the anecdotes here is, when at the beginning of my writing career somebody asked me what genres I wrote in, I would answer "fiction and non-fiction," often adding, "But not a memoir!"

The vehemence of this statement seemed to surprise people. They would look at me strangely or try to nod when I expressed how hard writing a memoir would be. They didn't mind one way or another.

At some point, which I described in my book *Cheerleading for Writers*, I realized that the person urging me to write a memoir was myself (see the excerpt at the end of this chapter). I even wrote various essays on my website, and my very first book, a novel based on the story of my father, was written from the first person and sounded like a memoir.

But I was still afraid to write a whole book as a memoir. I tried to do so, and offered to write a memoir essay collection with a friend, mixing her stories and mine. She agreed, and permitted me to choose from any of the life stories she had written and published along with those of other writers on a blog devoted to the memories of those who were young in the middle of the twentieth century[6]. I started reading through her and my blog posts and then switched to other projects, making little progress on our story collection.

Now, having openly embarked on memoir writing, and read more on the topic, I realize that one of the reasons I stopped might have been the following. The working title of the essay collection was *Everywhere at Home*, and I had intended to show that wherever you are in the world, you can feel at home there. I had a strong desire to concentrate on positivity, on great memories, and in a way, I was attempting to reject anything negative. But one can't write a memoir that deals with only those things that have met or exceeded their preferences.

The bestselling memoir writer Rachael Herron emphasizes this truth passionately in her acclaimed book

---

[6] https://www.timegoesby.net/elderstorytelling/marcy-belson/

Fast-Draft Your Memoir and says, "We want to hear how people failed, how they tried, how they made mistakes, and how they survived in spite of their imperfections. Your readers want to read how you struggled, failed, and got back up. That's all we want. Show your reader the worst of you, and they'll believe the best. (Caution: the reverse is also true.) We want to see your broken places and compare them to our own cracks and mended joints."

Today, I don't reject what I don't like as often as I did before, even if this urge still appears from time to time.

The other reason for my resistance towards writing a memoir might have been my idea that I should write it chronologically. And, as I mentioned above in the chapter about chronology, there is no way I could do that.

Again, learning the craft of writing a memoir from Rachael Herron and many others (some of my favorites are listed in "Further Reading"), I discovered that it is not necessary. There is another type of memoir that covers topics rather than time. This book is topic-based. It is all about dealing with various health challenges and healing myself in the process.

But I still can't shake the feeling that it is not a one-hundred-percent memoir. Many of the words coming out of my head and fingertips have much more to do with the present moment, and my present view of the past. As mentioned above, my memories are merely pictures made from the perspective of my current self; the latter always evolving, in often unpredictable ways.

In this book, you will find I use phrases like "this morning," "a few minutes ago," "right now," or other such references to recently experienced moments that are quite close to the present moment, as in the moment when I put these words to the page.

For you as a reader, and my future self during the review of the book and other possible occasions, the moments conveyed by such words will be in the past. But at this moment, right now, they are generated by the present. The word "memoir," however, to my mind at least, points to a time further back than in the moments when the book was written.

[This is also mirrored by the various updates and side-notes added during the multiple revisions of this book, indicated by square brackets. These changes show that neither my health conditions nor my experience of turning them into fun games is static, and that they will be changing, in often surprising ways, for as long as I live.]

Another reason is that some chapters of this book might sound like a self-help book. I emphasize several times that these are just my experiences, and I don't recommend you copy what I did or try the diets I am following, but in terms of turning my life into games and the three approaches I tap into to do so, then, yes, I recommend that with all my heart.

These are two reasons for me calling this book "*Almost* a Memoir."

And here is another reason, which I mentioned in the introduction.

I can't say which I love reading more: fiction or non-fiction. Currently, I combine reading a bit of fiction with a bit of non-fiction. It rarely occurs that I read only fiction or only non-fiction books on any one day. In most cases, it is a colorful combination of different genres and styles every day.

And then, this idea of the parable. It is simply brilliant! In it, you don't have to preach what you want to communicate and teach, but instead, you can show the possible doubts that can arise while learning about your method, idea, or a lesson learned. You can show empathy in a parable so much better than stating in your non-fiction book, "I know how it feels."

A memoir comes close to a parable too, in that you can show how you struggled before you could stand up, or even how you still struggle from time to time, as I do, and as most of us do, but are able to get up and get going again.

So, here is how I see this book: I am exploring myself as the main character of my own parable. Well, we are all the protagonists of our own lives. You are in yours, and I am in mine.

But I will still call on the help of Vivi, (fictitious) Jen, and Luca occasionally, and tell you what I had in mind for them in various situations. The characters of any book have bits of the writer in them, and this is true for Vivi, Jen, and Luca too. These three, along with the real characters in my life who carry and inspire me, will hopefully make the picture of my path complete, and help you to see your own more clearly.

Excerpt from *Cheerleading for Writers*:

I started telling my friends, "I will never write memoirs. That is simply not me!"

In reply, they shrugged, a bit surprised at my exclamation, as none of them had asked whether I wanted to write a memoir. But I kept repeating it, even when somebody was only asking me what genres I wrote in. Eventually, the ever-returning and threatening statement, "But not memoirs!" made me frown. If nobody required me to write one, why did I say "no" aloud?

After some searching and contemplation, I recalled when this idea of "Memoirs-are-not-for-me" formed for the first time. I'd once found a long article about memoirs and eagerly read every word of it. Somewhere in the middle, my thoughts had shouted, *No, this is too complicated. Memoirs are not for me. They are too conflicting and will stir too much worry in me and those I am writing about!*

From that moment, I kept repeating this statement to myself and others, "Memoirs are not for me! I am writing only in one genre!"

The truth, however, was different.

The truth was that my first and second books, which I wrote and published before this strange internal battle about memoirs commenced, were of very different genres. I wasn't writing in one genre, to begin with.

My blog posts, on the other hand, still had another unique shape. I avoided thinking about their "shapes" as genres. I still had this idea that I had to and wanted to stick with one style.

But why was I so often thinking of memoirs, when I supposedly write only fiction? Why was I answering this question with a "no," that no one was even asking? Who was asking me to write a memoir?

As I relaxed, took a step back and looked at it, I had the answer. *I* was the one who wanted to write a memoir. And the fact was that I was already doing it. I did it on my blog and also in my very first book, *The Truth About Family*, which I based on the true story of my father. I wrote this book in the first person as if my dad had written his very own memoir.

6. Anthropology

This book, and my life really, is a journey of study, a journey of learning. Sometimes a reluctant one that I feel is imposed on me by the ever-changing and surprising nature of life, but at other times, and I hope more and more often, a voluntary, open, and curious one.

My father was a scientist, as was my mother. My father tried to lure my sister into physics, because it was his subject and he loved it, but he never managed to. He didn't have time to try it with me, but his early death and me missing him somehow did so in his place.

I studied semiconductor physics, as he did.

Nowadays, I am interested in anthropology in layman and popular terms, but do not aspire for a Ph.D. in the subject, like I have in electrical engineering.

Here is one of the shortest and one of the most telling definitions of anthropology:

"Anthropology is the study of the human species, from DNA to language." — Cameron M. Smith, *Anthropology For Dummies*

Cameron Smith quotes the anthropologist Clyde Kluckhohn, who in 1949 "published 'Mirror for Man,' an introduction to the study of anthropology, the study of humanity (anthro meaning 'of humanity' and logy meaning 'the study of')."

Smith claims the following, "Kluckhohn's words still ring true: 'Anthropology holds up a great mirror to man and lets him look at himself in his infinite variety.'" — Cameron M. Smith, *Anthropology For Dummies*

Today, I am sometimes surprised by how long it took me to become interested in this amazing and essential science.

After all, I am human, and anthropology is the multi-dimensional scientific discipline of studying humanity in its many aspects.

But the best thing about it is that anthropology today is non-judgmental.

"One foundation of anthropology is the *comparative approach*, in which cultures aren't compared to one another in terms of which is better than the other but rather in an attempt to understand how and why they differ as well as share commonalities. This method is also known as *cultural relativism*, an approach that rejects making moral judgments about different kinds of humanity and simply examines each relative to its own unique origins and history." — Cameron M. Smith, *Anthropology For Dummies*

I tried to understand myself for many years. There seemed to be so many strange things about me when I compared myself to others. Sometimes, I even wondered if I was human. Or maybe a human with a "defect." I couldn't have children when my husband and I tried to; I couldn't eat the same things others did. I felt so different from everyone else. I rarely fit in any visible grouping, and when I did, for example the "gluten-intolerant group," it would be an unfavourable one, and it would still be an imperfect fit; having all those strange reactions to gluten, and all.

There always seemed to be something wrong. Even when my biggest dreams came true (such as having a family), I seemed to be unhappy. I couldn't believe that my intolerances or other challenges were the only reasons. I must have been doing something wrong, which probably also lead to all the issues with my health. Even until recently, I was convinced that I must have a single physical condition that was responsible for all the others: my multiple food intolerances, low blood count, eye condition, osteoarthritis, my mild allergies, high sensitivity to perfume, and anything else that I might have forgotten or not discovered yet.

Over the years, I bought and read many self-help books, and none of them seemed to give me a plausible answer to why I was, in my opinion, screwed up and hopeless, until I read the book *Being Here* by the award-winning authors, and my now dear friends, Ariel and Shya Kane.

While reading this book, I, for the first time, was able to question whether my life and myself were screwed up, or whether I simply judged them that way.

With time, I learned and experienced the three revealing principles of their anthropological approach.

First, I realized that if I resisted something or tried to get rid of something – a thought, a habit, a person, a task, experience of pain, or anything else – I didn't get rid of it at all. This person, feeling, or thing just kept on sticking around, dominated my life, and often became overwhelming.

Then, I learned that I couldn't be anywhere else or anyone else or feel any differently at any given moment – I could only be who and how I was (or wasn't), whether I liked it or not. And whether I judged my situation or not.

Finally, anything that I allowed to be in any given moment exactly as it was without judging or trying to change it completed itself in an instant, including my suffering.

As I read Ariel and Shya's books and articles, listened to their *Being Here* internet radio show, and participated in their live seminars, I experienced what it meant to let myself and others be just as we were. I discovered the possibility to breathe and experience my life moment by moment, completely and freely.

I am still in awe of the simplicity and fantastic effect of one of their ideas.

They suggest that each of us studies oneself as a culture of one.

"Practice your anthropological approach. Pretend you're a scientist observing a culture of one — yourself. The trick is not to judge what you see but to neutrally observe how you function, including your thought processes. Awareness and kindness are key." — Ariel and Shya Kane, *How to Have A Match Made in Heaven*

That was one of the biggest and most amazing discoveries of my life, as well as an immense blessing.

It opened the possibility for me to relax and have fun in my life. It also paved the way for me to learn about two other amazing approaches, which I unknowingly already applied. Along with awareness, these approaches became the fantastic toolset I use to navigate my life however it may turn out, with more engagement and joy than I ever had before.

Learning from Ariel and Shya Kane and their anthropological approach to living in the moment, I finally discovered the one physical condition that explained all the issues I have with my health. I found it in the sequel to *Being Here*, which has the beautiful and apt title *Being Here...Too*:

"Everyone has a terminal illness – it's called life. None of us know how long our lives are going to be. It's so easy to put off doing the things you want, and doing the things that need to be done." — Ariel and Shya Kane, *Being Here...Too*

It is inspiring to see how these two, and other fantastic people devoting their work to empowering others, "go about [their lives] with urgency as if this day could be [their] last." — Ariel and Shya Kane, *Being Here...Too*

And here is another inspiring quote by Ariel and Shya Kane that concludes wonderfully the two above, and which I already quoted in my very first book about turning life into fun games, *5 Minute Perseverance Game*:

"Life is fleeting. If you have the idea you want to do something, you should go for it." — Ariel and Shya Kane

7. Kaizen

The other amazing tool I apply today and learn to use more and more, and which helped me tremendously in my life, is kaizen.

I read about kaizen for the first time in British journalist and best-selling author Helen Russell's fun and inspiring book, *Leap Year*. In it Russell interviewed Dr. Robert Maurer[7], Director of Behavioral Sciences for the Family Practice Residency Program at Santa Monica, UCLA Medical Center, and a faculty member at the UCLA School of Medicine.

I was intrigued by the idea of small steps toward continuous improvement, and the effortlessness of those small steps.

I searched for kaizen on one of the largest online bookstores. The first book that appeared and seemed to be most purchased and most liked was *One Small Step Can Change Your Life*, written by the person Helen Russell had interviewed: Robert Maurer. He had also written several other popular books on small steps and kaizen, including *Mastering Fear* and *The Spirit of Kaizen*.

---

[7] http://www.scienceofexcellence.com/ and http://www.scienceofexcellence.com/one-small-step-can-change-your-life-book.php

Here are a few quotes by Robert Maurer about kaizen:

"Kaizen is as much a philosophy or belief system as it is a strategy for success in changing or enhancing some behavior."

"Kaizen is an ancient philosophy captured in this powerful statement from the Tao Te Ching: 'The journey of a thousand miles begins with a single step.'"

"Kaizen has two definitions:

- using very small steps to improve a habit, a process, or product

- using very small moments to inspire new products and inventions" — Robert Maurer, *One Small Step Can Change Your Life*

In *One Small Step Can Change Your Life*, Robert Maurer shows "how easy change can be when the brain's preference for change is honored."

Robert Maurer formulated six strategies for applying kaizen on a personal level.

"The succeeding chapters are devoted to the personal application of kaizen and encompass six different strategies. These strategies include:

- asking small questions to dispel fear and inspire creativity

- thinking small thoughts to develop new skills and habits — without moving a muscle

- taking small actions that guarantee success

- solving small problems, even when you're faced with an overwhelming crisis

- bestowing small rewards to yourself or others to produce the best results

- recognizing the small but crucial moments that everyone else ignores." — Robert Maurer, *One Small Step Can Change Your Life*

That says it all. In the spirit of kaizen, we can break anything, either a challenge or a task or whatever we are paying attention to, down into small and effortless steps. And we give each of these small bits our full attention, which is easy if the task is small enough to solve with little effort.

In Robert Maurer's book, I read one of the most enlightening, memorable, and empowering, as well as perspective-changing, statements about the steps we try to make toward our goals.

"Even the small signs that you are resisting the small step are an indication that the step is too big." — Robert Maurer, *One Small Step Can Change Your Life*

From Ariel and Shya Kane, I learned that when I tried to get something over with, I was resisting it. But "what you resist persists, grows stronger, and dominates your life." — Ariel and Shya Kane, *Working on Yourself Doesn't Work*

And so it was with all the conditions I had. The more I resisted and didn't want to have them, the stronger their effects on me became. Or, at the very least, I experienced them in a much stronger way.

However, if I approached them the kaizen way, taking one little step that was doable where I was at that moment and with what I had at hand (including the pain I experienced), and if I tackled just a tiny bit of a single challenge at a time, then my whole situation ceased to feel overwhelming.

So, instead of trying to reach the state I wanted to achieve in one go, and being daunted by the immense scale of the task, I started behaving as athletes do when they train for the big win. "Just as a record-setting marathon runner will continue to search out ways to shave another second off his or her best time, you can seek out strategies to constantly sharpen your life's game." — Robert Maurer, *One Small Step Can Change Your Life*

This awareness was utterly rewarding.

You might wonder why I am introducing you to techniques you may not have heard of before. The use of kaizen, anthropology, and non-judgmental seeing, described above, and the tool I will address in the next chapter, will be obvious throughout the book. I describe them here so that you know what I use in my life, and what permits me to cope with my health issues gamefully, and to approach healing in a light and joyful way whenever possible.

And now, let's get to the last tool.

8. Gamification

Awareness of the present moment and living life to the full embrace the possibility of enjoying life. The joy to breathe, the joy to be able to explore, the joy to be challenged.

As children, we are very wise. We are naturally curious. But as we get older, this curiosity is replaced by a yearning for comfort.

Complaints are pretty comfortable, but they are not fun. Not at all.

So what can we do?

OK, first of all, do not judge the situation. It's rainy now, my joints are complaining, and I can't eat what I would prefer (or rather *think* that I would prefer), like some sweets or something.

But wait a second. Something else is there too. I am not hungry; my stomach feels comfortable; there is no pain. I am sitting in a warm room in front of my computer and am doing one of the best things in the world: I am writing a book. And besides this, I just took a sip of my favorite drink, espresso, followed by what is deemed healthy but I can admit to also loving – still water.

So life shows up as it does, and I can be aware of it, and approach it one little step at a time: like taking in all that is there, both preferable and not, writing a word at a time, and sipping my espresso and water one bit at a time.

But there is something else we need to be aware of. And that is appreciation.

This idea might surprise you, but I mean appreciating the challenges life poses, in a fun way. Through the awareness that we can add fun elements to those challenges, in order to appreciate the small steps we have taken to master them. Please note that by "master" I don't mean "overcome," as that would be a form of resistance, but rather navigating them, whatever the "weather."

And how can we achieve that appreciation?

By being aware of what makes us curious, what is fun, like games, for example. We don't need to add drama to what we do. Instead, we can turn anything in our lives into fun games.

That was one of the most rewarding and fun discoveries I had. Turning my life into games helped me maintain my sense of humor, even in situations that many people would find challenging.

Here is an idea, which I tested and enjoyed many times since I started turning my life into fun games. I remembered multiple times when I wanted to entertain my children while motivating them to do what needed to be done in a fun way. I thought of how I had ideas for making challenges fun and came up with small fun rewards, as many parents nowadays do.

Just in the spirit of Mary Poppins, who sang in her famous song "A Spoonful of Sugar," the following enlightening words:

"In ev'ry job that must be done

There is an element of fun

You find the fun and snap!

The job's a game."

Couldn't I be doing the same for myself? Of course, I could! So I asked myself, how could I make any of the goals in the projects and activities I was up to as enticing as a quest in a game? And how could I reward myself for every step taken on the way, especially the small ones? Not material (or at least not expensive), but fun rewards?

I realized that for me, it was by giving myself points (usually a tally on a scrap of paper), or stars and badges, by recording them in a weekly calendar or keeping a list of each task completed during the day, as I accomplished them. Or celebrating a page typed or edited with a colorful, glittery sticker on that page as soon as it was done. Thus, I used gameful and playful elements to appreciate what I did during the day. I also had modified ways of approaching different tasks. For example, I danced while doing some of them, or gave myself the challenge of exercising before doing an activity I considered a reward.

I wouldn't be the first to bring fun game elements into real-life activities. There is a whole field of science and even industry, or art. This art of bringing fun elements from games into real-life situations is called gamification[8].

And when I applied it to myself, I discovered there was also a need for awareness (anthropological, non-judgmental seeing) and progress in small steps (kaizen).

As a result, I now own the ultimate tool, like those early versions of Swiss Army Knives (for example, the "The Soldier Knife model 1890 had a spear point blade, reamer, can-opener, screwdriver and grips made out of oak wood scales (handles) that were treated with

---

[8] Gamification is "the use of game design elements in non-game contexts" — Deterding, S., Dixon, D., Khaled, R., & Nacke, L. (2011). From game design elements to gamefulness: defining gamification. In Proceedings of the 15th international academic MindTrek conference: Envisioning future media environments (pp. 9-15). ACM.
(https://www.researchgate.net/publication/230854710_From_Game_Design_Elements_to_Gamefulness_Defining_Gamification)

rapeseed oil for greater toughness and water-repellency, which made them black in color." – Wikipedia[9]).

I call this special "Swiss Army Knife" for turning my life into games Self-Gamification.

---

[9] "The Swiss Army knife is a pocketknife or multi-tool manufactured by Victorinox (and up to 2005 also by Wenger SA). The term 'Swiss Army knife' was coined by American soldiers after World War II due to the difficulty they had in pronouncing 'Offiziersmesser,' the German name (lit. 'officer's knife')." — Wikipedia (https://en.wikipedia.org/wiki/Swiss_Army_knife)

9. Self-Gamification

So what is this special "Swiss Army Knife"? The three-in-one tool I remind myself I have as often as I can, on any hike through my life, be it in a calm "rural" area with no bumps or rush, or in a high-paced "city" of appointments and requests that life poses, in its various and ever-surprising ways?

I call this tool Self-Gamification, which is the art of turning our lives into fun games. And it's not only an art; each of the component tools is a product of the art and wisdom collected and shared by many people, in their unique way.

But this Self-Gamification is also a synergy of three approaches coming together and supporting each other. And it is also a possibility.

Isn't it amazing to know that we can turn anything, any challenge, however big or daunting into a fun game? I tested this theory many times, and it became a practice. Even before I formulated it. I test it today again and again. Both because I enjoy it, and also to find out what else is possible without pressure or effort, and instead with fun and enjoyment.

This tool, art, and possibility embraces three skill-sets, just like a simple Swiss Army Knife can help to cut, open a can, and to repair something with an in-built screw-driver, for example.

Here is another analogy I bring up often to show how these three approaches, methods, and philosophies create a fantastic synergy. This synergy has its foundation in awareness (non-judgmental, anthropological seeing and engaging), and progresses one brick (small-step) at a time, to build a beautiful and fun (gameful) house that we enjoy being in.

Thus, the three skills needed to result in what I call Self-Gamification are the ones I described in the three previous chapters. And they unfold as follows.

First of all, it is to see ourselves, the world around us, and the thought processes arising both from inside and from our interaction with the world, non-judgmentally, just like an anthropologist would do while studying an utterly interesting for him or her culture.

Already at this stage, we can play a game:

"You can create a game where you pretend you are a scientist or an anthropologist discovering the way that a particular culture functions or operates." — Ariel and Shya Kane, *Working on Yourself Doesn't Work*

The second is to be able to identify and take the smallest, most effortless step in the direction we want to move, that is toward our dreams and goals, the kaizen way.

And the third is to perform and appreciate each step in a fun way. It is also the readiness to learn from anything that appears gameful or playful to each of us. The readiness to learn from anyone who deals with games, and most of all, from game designers and players, and get inspired by them.

These three skill sets are interconnected, reinforce each other, and enable us to see what we do or what we are up to as a game, of which *we are both the designers and the players.*

Awareness is the primary component and the basis for their synergy. You can't identify the next step or what is fun for you without being aware of what's going on inside and outside you and how these two worlds interact.

Thus, awareness opens the door to this possibility, and reveals this three-in-one tool; this amazing "Swiss Army Knife" that allows me to carve something I enjoy bit by bit, like a beautiful wooden sculpture, while helping to do something else, for example, nourish myself, using the other two parts of the knife.

That was about the base, the foundation, of the sculpture I am creating here with this book.

I will carve the rest out of the old and seasoned wood of memories, adding the wisdom of precious stones I had the honor to touch upon as I grew up, and the newer, sparkling glitter of experiences I have right now. All of them will be "touched" by the three-in-one tool of Self-Gamification.

10. Healing

The possibilities that studying myself as an anthropologist would a culture, or a game-designer the players of his/her games and by that finding ways to modify the game design so that the players enjoy it — the game and life, really — offer, never fail to amaze me.

Recently I discovered that I have osteoarthritis, and that this was responsible for the discomfort I experienced, and my reduced participation in the daily yoga-workout game (as I like calling it) I had previously enjoyed for over half a year. I then understood that labeling myself lazy for not working out was not helpful, as laziness wasn't the core reason.

[A side-note: "Osteoarthritis is the most common form of arthritis, affecting millions of people worldwide. It occurs when the protective cartilage that cushions the ends of your bones wears down over time. Although osteoarthritis can damage any joint, the disorder most commonly affects joints in your hands, knees, hips and spine." — Mayo Clinic[10]]

Shortly after, I realized something that might appear quite strange at first.

---

[10] https://www.mayoclinic.org/diseases-conditions/osteoarthritis/symptoms-causes/syc-20351925

I became aware that every time I told someone about my hurting joints and they said, "Get well soon," I had the urge to answer (or even scream), "I can't get well! The internet says there's no cure for it!"

Of course, I wanted others to wish me well. *I* wanted me to be well! Very much so. But still, there was this resistance.

Fortunately, I didn't follow this urge to scream and thanked the well-wishers as best I could, confused by my resisting feeling inside.

When I became aware of it without judging, I was very surprised about my apparent anger when others wished me to get well soon. It seemed as though I wanted to keep the pain around, to justify the suffering.

Wow, that discovery was very interesting. Didn't I complain about *not* enjoying the pain and hating the suffering? I did, but when the wishes went in the same direction, for the suffering to be removed and me to be free from pain, I resisted? Hm.

What could have been the reason for that? Did I have to search for those reasons?

Maybe something along with the formula:

"Nothing is more desirable than to be released from an affliction, but nothing is more frightening than to be divested of a crutch." — James Baldwin quoted in *Maybe You Should Talk to Someone* by Lori Gottlieb

To read this quote, sounding like a universal truth, was a relief. So, many felt as I did. But, of course, the reasons could be different for every one of us, and they could be multiple.

Remarkably, anthropologists, don't look for reasons. The awareness is enough to undo the knot.

Awareness occurs when we observe ourselves non-judgmentally. Ariel and Shya Kane, whose work I quote often, define awareness as follows:

"A nonjudgmental, non-preferential seeing. It's an objective, noncritical witnessing of the nature or what we call the 'isness' of any particular circumstance or situation. It can be described as an ongoing process in which you are bringing yourself back to the moment, rather than complaining silently about how you would prefer this moment to be." — Ariel and Shya Kane, *Practical Enlightenment*

So to be aware, I didn't have to do anything complex or difficult. All I needed to do was to look around and observe. This observation included seeing and listening without validating what I saw or heard. It was about discovering anew without comparing to what I already knew. Such seeing and listening brought to any moment a newly experienced crispness and freshness.

That also applied to my health conditions. Seeing myself non-judgmentally, revealed that I was upset about my situation. Again, the reasons for that might have been multiple. But the fact was, I was upset. It was like bringing light into a dark room. Until then, I lived through the upset, but I didn't see it non-judgmentally and didn't clearly and honestly say (illuminated), "Huh, I am upset!"

That realization brought the next question, though. What did being upset mean, anyway? I searched online and found the following definition for being upset. We are then "unhappy, disappointed, or worried." — Oxford Dictionaries[11]

What could the reasons be for being unhappy, disappointed, and worried? It was, of course, hard to grasp all possible ones. I did realize that. But was there perhaps one main source for them? Or one that is true for many who are upset? Here is what Robert Maurer said on that:

"Do all upsets come from fear? We don't know for sure. However, based on the research, I suggest that this is the most useful way of looking at them." — Robert Maurer, *Mastering Fear*

I could see now that the emotions I had when somebody wished me to get well were most probably the fear about what could happen if this pain went away. What would

---

[11] https://en.oxforddictionaries.com/definition/upset

happen then, was unknown to me. I knew the pain. I didn't like it, but I had got to know it, at least some of its facets. But the unknown was scary. Would feeling better mean that I would be able, and have to, move more, do more? What if that caused even more pain?

Nobody could answer these questions for me, and nobody can know that for sure. So why think it?

Well, I couldn't stop my thoughts from appearing and my mind from fretting. And as soon as these thoughts were there, the moment was gone.

But I could start being curious in the next moment, about what would be the next, closest step to take.

I could also see those thoughts as an indicator, a little light-emitting diode, or a blue light and a loud siren, going off when something was amiss when a part of my brain wanted to draw attention to the fact that action was needed.

When I look non-judgmentally now at how I felt and thought then, I realize that in those moments of resistance when my little red lamp (or the big blue light with a siren) went off, I was afraid that healing would cause more pain. I see now how strange and paradoxical that sounds. I am also aware now that I was upset about not being able to get rid of the pain completely. I felt like my body was "fooling me" with only partial healing.

After all, my body was sending alarm signals more and more often as I aged, which seemed to me like my healing attempts didn't work. Or they worked only temporarily.

Was such a temporary relief worth it if the pain would inevitably come back someday, and most likely in an unexpected form? Shouldn't I just carry on with the pain and try to get used to it, or get some pain-killers to put the alarm system off? Why care about the cause if there will just be another someday anyway?

A sudden realization hit me as a series of photographs in time; memories flashing through my mind in answer to these questions. First, of my parents taking care of my cuts, scratches, and blisters, and then of me helping my children with theirs.

Here is what I became aware of through this slide show of memories: When we have an open wound, we clean it, put some balm on it, and cover it if necessary with a plaster or a band-aid, all aimed at helping our bodies to heal the wound. We don't carry on playing in the mud and putting more dirt on it if the pain increases. We clean it up and take gentle care of it.

If we can't do it ourselves, we ask for the help of a professional. But we do something to help our bodies to heal. And... to live.

At some point, we won't be able to heal anymore. But until then, we can support ourselves in healing, both physically and emotionally.

Others do wish that for us often, with all their hearts.

As I unveiled that unsolved resistance and became aware of what the real name of the health navigation game is, namely, the Healing Game along with the Play and Have Fun Game, I realized that I wish that not only for all my loved ones, and to all people in general, but I wish it for myself as well.

So that is another aspect of the sculpture I am creating here with this book. The following stories will show how I learned to help myself to heal every time I needed to, and how I also gradually let others support my healing.

11. My Body

I don't remember hating my body, although I might have complained about it, or was embarrassed when somebody made a compliment. Now, I think I was just confused by the state of it. If somebody complimented me on my shape, I wondered if they were being honest, and instead, if I was too curvy with too many problem zones. If someone congratulated me on my eyes, I wondered if my nose was too bent. If someone said I was slim, I wondered if I was too skinny.

And certainly, when told that I was skinny, overweight, or something about my posture, which all happened, I wondered when the time would come that nobody would comment on my body, so that I could go about my day without noticing it.

It is strange to see that now. Yes, I rarely had strong feelings about my body in the past.

For the most part, I ignored it. Or I tried to. Even hearing and nodding in agreement to advice not to ignore my body, but to value it, didn't help for long. After some half-hearted attempt to take care of it somehow, I would go back to paying no attention at all. And I did so for as long as I could.

I was confused when my attention was drawn to it. I didn't know what to do and how to behave.

But the biggest confusion came when my body drew my attention to it all by itself. And it did so more and more often with time.

I started asking myself all kinds of disturbing questions I couldn't answer. While doing sports, my muscles began aching right after I started exercising, and I was quickly out of breath. Was it normal to feel that way? Wasn't I supposed to become tired a bit later? Maybe I wasn't fit enough. Why did I get tired anyway, when I had so much fun in the beginning before all the aching commenced? Why did I faint in front of everyone at school? What would happen the next day? Why did I get that cramp again even though I increased my intake of magnesium supplements, and why did my stomach hurt?

All through that chat in my head over the years and then attempt to shrug off the signals, my body still made sure to interrupt my taking it for granted every once in a while. As you see from the incomplete and chaotic collection of questions above, which arose from any new, or forgotten and, thus, unknown signal from my body, especially when it was discomforting, the main questions were "What's wrong?" and "Why is this happening to me?"

Only nowadays, with the Self-Gamification tools under my belt, do I start asking, "Why not?", "How can I gamefully master this new challenging level?"

Nowadays, I try not to ignore my body as soon as my "wounds" heal, and the pain recedes. It isn't often possible, now that my joints remind me of their existence in almost every moment. But, thanks to this condition, I rarely take the absence of pain for granted anymore. I notice it and am amazed by it. At first, the absence of pain also confused me, and I would wonder what was happening. I observed myself deciding, "Now, it's gone." And be taken by surprise when it reappeared shortly after.

I realize now more and more often that pain or the experience of pain, as well as its absence, are just sensations, and I can also experience them as such, without labeling them as "bad" or "painful" and "good" or "not painful." On the other hand, I am a human being who uses speech and labels to describe something. So labeling them as painful and hurtful is not bad either, I just do it.

The trick is not to judge all the thoughts appearing in my mind but to study them as a scientist and as each game designer, creating the best and most enjoyable games for her player, myself.

Jane McGonigal, in her acclaimed book *SuperBetter*, quotes a number of studies that show games can reduce the experience of pain. She especially addresses the enjoyment of playing the game. When you enjoy doing something, you don't notice and experience pain as drastically as you did before practicing the fun activity.

She described how researchers found that burn victims paid less attention to their pain when they played a video game *Snow World*. The patients were aware of their injuries and experienced pain during wound care, but they focused their attention on playing the game. As a result, they didn't have to receive strong medicine, usually morphine, to alleviate "the most intense and prolonged pain a human being can experience." — Jane McGonigal, *SuperBetter*

The following passages in Jane McGonigal's book were eye-opening for me:

"In scientific papers describing the game's positive impacts, *Snow World*'s inventors, Dr. Hunter Hoffman and Dr. David Patterson, attribute its success to a well-established psychological phenomenon: *the spotlight theory of attention.*

"According to this theory, human attention is like a spotlight. Your brain can process and absorb only a limited amount of new information at any given moment. So you focus on one source of information at a time, ignoring everything else. As a result, information everywhere competes constantly for your brain's attention—sights, sounds, tastes, smells, thoughts, and physical sensations.

"What does this have to do with pain? The signals from your nerves that cause pain are just one of many competing streams of information. It's a particularly compelling stream. Your nerves are sending signals to your brain to let you know that you're injured—which is pretty important information! It makes perfect sense that without conscious intervention, you'd be more likely to focus your attention spotlight on these pain signals than just about any other source of information.

"But you're not powerless against pain signals. In fact, if you learn to control your attention spotlight, you can actually stop your brain from spending its limited processing resources on pain signals from your nerves."

She concludes with the following:

"If you don't want your brain to pay attention to pain signals, give it something else to pay attention to instead." — Jane McGonigal, *SuperBetter*

Now I understand why writing has such a healing effect on me. I love writing. Among other things, it enlightens me. It is one of the most amazing experiences I have in my life, and which I want to do again and again with all my heart. But as for many writers, writing can still appear daunting to me. From time to time my brain still pictures the creative and writing processes as tedious and tiring and long. Awareness helps me recognize from moment to moment that this dynamic in my thought processes is the beautiful effect of creativity. Writing awakens and inspires me, and it draws as well as sharpens my attention.

So when I type these words, I do notice the joints in my fingers, but this feeling is not as unsettling as it is when my brain is freed from the engaging activity of writing and has enough space to create worries or magnify the experience of pain. Thus, if I give my brain a fun challenge, it is less able to fill itself with worries.

We will talk about fun a bit later, but for now, having the tools of awareness, small steps, and the lightness and fun elements that games provide, let's consider this sample of humanity, me, and the stories of that "specimen" getting ill and healing herself, in some detail.

12. Food Intolerance

"A food intolerance, or a food sensitivity occurs when a person has difficulty digesting a particular food." — AAAAI (AAAAI is American Academy of Allergy Asthma & Immunology)[12]

If the story about the parable started with a writing competition, then the story of my awareness about my food intolerances — probably my most complex chronic condition — started with a party. Here there is also a backstory, but more on that later.

It was the end of February 2008 and my sister-in-law's thirtieth birthday party (Oh, that's why my fictitious character Vivi's sister was celebrating her thirtieth as well! How did I not see that parallel before?! Clever, tricky mind. ;)). I don't remember the whole party clearly, although I remember it was great. But strangely, I remember the moment I discovered that the word "intolerance" could be applied to describe not only a character's fault, but also the way a human body may react to food.

I was sitting not far from a table with a wide range of cakes, facing it. Next to me, sat my mother-in-law. I

---

[12] https://www.aaaai.org/conditions-and-treatments/conditions-dictionary/food-intolerance

don't remember what we chatted about, but at some point, I noticed that she held her hand to her stomach. I either did it too or wanted to, because I had bad heartburn and stomach pain.

I don't remember how, but I must have asked her which cake she ate. She pointed, if I remember correctly, at a plum tart on the table in front of us. Just before joining her (or her joining me), I had eaten the same thing.

I also don't remember if I asked her about the pain in her stomach. But at some point, she told me that she should have avoided the tart because of the histamine intolerance doctors had told her she had, but she couldn't resist eating it.

I had no idea what histamine was, let alone the fact that it could or could not be tolerated.

[A side-note: Histamine is "a compound which is released by cells in response to injury and in allergic and inflammatory reactions, causing contraction of smooth muscle and dilation of capillaries." — Lexico[13]. And "histamine intolerance occurs when there is a buildup of histamine in the body. Drugs, medical conditions, the environment, nutritional deficiencies, and diet can lead to histamine intolerance." — Medical News Today[14]]

---

[13] https://www.lexico.com/en/definition/histamine
[14] https://www.medicalnewstoday.com/articles/322543

I must have repeated that phrase "histamine intolerance" with a question mark on my face, because my mom-in-law explained to me what histamine was, and why some human bodies cannot tolerate it.

Human bodies can misinterpret normal and even healthy food (I mean, plums have plenty of vitamins, even in baked form and even covered with sugar, right?) and think it is bad and then act strangely. Was my body doing the same?

I must have asked my mom-in-law that question out loud because she urged me to go to my doctor about it.

Seeing a doctor, however, especially my physician at that time, was what I dreaded most of all. The next two chapters will explain why.

13. The Dentist

I loved doctors as a child. Especially dentists. We had a family friend who was a dentist, and he treated all of us. My sister dreaded any dentist, including him. But I loved him, because he was funny, and because he gave me discarded drills and little boxes. I treated many of my dolls for caries. I even tried to do the same with my big sister. Yes, the one who dreaded dentists. (I have only one sister.) Imagine being chased around by your eight-and-a-half years younger sibling to treat your teeth with some broken and discarded tooth-drill. That was her destiny over forty years ago, which she managed to escape.

Being a big fan of our family friend and dentist, for a long time I even wanted to become a dentist myself, until my last deciduous (better known as milk) tooth was taken out. I was a teenager then and went to the clinic by myself. Our family friend and dentist was not working that day, or he had retired by that time, I don't quite remember, but I was to be taken care of by a young doctor, who seemed to be as nervous as I was. Or even more so.

He told me that I was his first patient to treat of the day, and if I remember correctly, it was his first day of treating someone on his own, that is without supervision by a senior colleague. And it was his first official day as a practicing dentist. I didn't quite know what that meant. I just noticed that this adult was so nervous that he looked like he was trembling.

Our uncle dentist usually took out my milk teeth (those that were more tricky and couldn't fall out or be taken out at home) easily, if I remember correctly with just a gloved hand and no tweezers. But I might be mistaken. In any case, he always made it look and feel so easy and painless.

But on that day with the young (and handsome, I must say) doctor, nothing seemed to be simple. He gave me an injection with anesthesia, but missed the point he'd wanted to get it. Then it happened once or twice again. Much of my face felt frozen after that. Then he took the tooth out, breaking it in the process. A small bit remained. He called a senior doctor for help, who finished the procedure.

I wasn't in much pain then, and I remember my feeling of curiosity and novelty. But there was also another thought there, which changed my desire to become a dentist entirely. I thought, if I became the dentist, then I would have to go through the same worry and terror as this guy. I would struggle to take out the teeth of some children and adults and risk hurting them. I wouldn't be able to avoid hurting them!

Then I recalled how mortified I was if I ever hurt my mom even slightly while cutting her nails, especially toenails. Now I realize that she must have asked my sister or me to do this because of her joint pain, but at that time I didn't connect the dots. She preferred me to cut her nails because, according to her, I had a light hand, and having the manicure and pedicure done by me (a very basic one) was even a pleasure. My mom was always sure that I would make an amazing dentist, physician, or surgeon.

But I was terrified of hurting anyone, even if it was for their own good, as doctors sometimes had to, and I apologized profusely and excessively anytime I suspected I may have hurt anyone. So the experience with the young, handsome dentist helped me to rule out medicine as a possible career completely and forever.

14. The Doctors

Even after my dentist experience, I didn't mind doctors or the occasional need to consult them.

We had some doctors and other medical personnel in our circle of family and friends.

We liked some more than others. But I didn't feel any strong reluctance towards medical personnel. That came later.

When I moved to Germany, and during the first ten years, there were several times I needed a doctor's intervention, after the initial health check. The biggest ones were a broken bone in my right foot, and later Bell's palsy on the right side of my face. The doctors couldn't find the reason for the Bell's palsy and assumed there was an infection of the main nerve on the right side of my face. They told me to watch out for and avoid cold wind on the right side of my face to prevent another Bell's palsy incident. They recommended that I look for other people who have experienced Bell's palsy and ask for their experiences. I found a colleague in another department who had had it eight times in total, less on one side and more on the other. She also recommended avoiding cold streams of air on both sides of the face, especially the affected one.

[A side-note: "Bell's palsy is a type of facial paralysis that results in an inability to control the facial muscles on the affected side. Symptoms can vary from mild to severe. They may include muscle twitching, weakness, or total loss of the ability to move one or rarely both sides of the face." — Wikipedia[15]]

The last two years or so before we moved to Denmark in 2008 were dominated by my stomach problems and frequent visits to my primary physician.

In the end my symptoms became so bad that I had to lie down after each meal and wait until the pain receded.

The worst time was during the meeting of an international working group, that took place in Tucson, Arizona. I had to flee the meeting pale and sick and stay in bed in my room until I felt better. The Sprite and other soda drinks recommended by the kind and helpful hotel personnel didn't help. My large collection of antacids, which I had expanded on in the United States, didn't help either. I got nauseous and sick on the flight back to Germany, sitting in the middle of the six-seat row of an intercontinental flight. It was mortifying. Until then I had only been sick once before whilst travelling, when much younger and having a forty-degree fever. Otherwise, I always took pride in never getting sick on any mode of transport and even bragged about how I could read or even write on a bus ride, even while standing.

---

15 https://en.wikipedia.org/wiki/Bell%27s_palsy

The party I mentioned in the chapter above about food intolerances took place four months before we moved to Denmark. It was the end of February 2008. In the two years before that, I was a frequent visitor to my doctor, and she had prescribed all kinds of medicine in an attempt to help me. I felt like I had a constant cold, with a runny nose for months, but no fever whatsoever.

When my mother-in-law suggested I go to my doctor and ask for tests to find out whether I had a food intolerance, I felt reluctant. I had the strong feeling that my doctor thought I was a hypochondriac and was trying to escape work. How could I prove to her that I loved my work and was considered a workaholic by many who knew me?

So, when I went to see my physician after the birthday party, I initially forgot everything I'd heard about histamine and other food intolerances from my mother-in-law.

That visit was completely different from all those before. I have several glimpses of memory from that visit and close to none for the multiple visits before that.

The first bit I remember is when the nurse showed me to one of the rooms and said, "Frau Doctor X will be with you in a minute." The "X" stands for my physician's name. I wouldn't remember her name anymore, if you asked me. But I did find it in my medical records from that time. But I am deliberately leaving her name out because it doesn't contribute to the story. You will see why in a minute.

What struck me that day is that I heard her name. I knew her name already, because there were two (if I remember correctly) doctors in that practice, and she was my physician, so I had used her name many times when asking for an appointment.

But on that day, when the nurse said her name, I looked up and felt a surprising feeling. It was like I realized for the first time that she was human like me.

Now I realize that my previous conversation with my mother-in-law must have triggered that effect somehow. I can vaguely remember her saying that doctors don't know everything and that they often need to guess because of the complexity of the human body and its reactions to various things.

Had you asked me, before that fateful visit, whether I thought my physician (or doctors in general) was human, I would have looked at you strangely and said, "Of course. What a strange question?!"

But even if I had always acknowledged her to be human, I hadn't considered her as human as I was — that is, permitted not to know everything and maybe even to make mistakes.

Maybe you have heard the phrase "gods in white" to describe doctors. There is even a German TV medical drama from 2017 with the same name ("Götter in Weiß"[16] in German).

That is exactly how I felt about doctors for most of my life, even with our family dentist. He seemed to never make mistakes. Doctors had to study for many years and work incredibly hard to become doctors, they knew everything and were better than everyone else. Their salaries were also higher due to the length and difficulty of their training, and the immensely complex art of their work, as I (and probably many others) thought. In my mind, there was always some distance between doctors and their patients, "mere mortals."

I realize now how strange that all sounds, but the trepidation I felt towards doctors for all those years could be the reason for such thought processes.

My feelings towards doctors changed considerably when we moved to Denmark. I was surprised and utterly pleased by two facts here. Nurses have as much (or sometimes even more) to say than doctors, and the patients (or their parents, if the patient is a child) are not only respected but also asked for their opinion.

I love telling how, during the necessary Cesarean delivery (C-section) of my daughter, I had a nurse there "only for my head." She put her arms around my head as I was lying on the operating table, placed her face

---

[16] "Götter in Weiß" —
https://www.imdb.com/title/tt6135514/

close to mine, and explained each step of the procedure before it occurred. The anesthetist made me laugh, and the surgeon thanked me for letting her help me bring my daughter into the world. Also, during the subsequent stay in hospital, my daughter and I got fantastic treatment, including getting meals that I could both tolerate and which tasted wonderful.

Unbeknownst to me, something must have changed in my perception of doctors when I talked to my mom-in-law at my sister-in-law's birthday party.

Because on the day when I visited my physician, I, first of all, heard her name. Then when she entered the room, I heard the nurse calling her by her first name. That diminished the distance I set between doctors and those like me even more.

And then what she said to me when I complained again that my stomach still ached after each meal, has stayed with me until now. She said, "I don't know what else to do. I have prescribed you everything there is. All the tests I ordered show normal values. I simply don't know how to help you further."

These words both shocked and amazed me. A doctor doesn't know what to do!? It sounded like she was almost asking me for help.

And strangely enough, that was the best thing she could have done to help me. Because suddenly, I remembered about the histamine intolerance.

I briefly recounted the incident at the birthday party and asked her whether I might have histamine intolerance.

Her face brightened, "Yes, it well might be a food intolerance. It is a relatively new field, and I am not an expert in it. But I have a colleague who researches a lot in this area, and he happens to support patients who are part of the Government Health Insurance System, as you are. I will transfer you to him." She called him on the spot and made an appointment for me.

I was dumbfounded. This doctor, whom I thought was being judgmental toward me, turned out to not only be utterly human, and without an immediate solution for everything, but also kind and helpful.

On that day, my exploration of what my body could and could not tolerate began.

15. An Alternative

My physician sent me to a doctor from another district. If I remember correctly, it was only a few days or a week until that other appointment.

That was another day I remember in detail. Or, at least, the visit with him. After taking a look at my medical documents and records from that time, I found the exact date: March 7, 2008.

In my memory, I had somehow superimposed several visits with him into one, and thought that everything — the test and his advice — took place on the same day. But checking those documents revealed that our interaction went on for at least a month. I am glad I kept all those recordings because it refreshes my memories and makes the picture, or the sculpture as I referred to this book in previous chapters, more distinct.

What I remember clearly is his warm smile and that he was kind and welcoming. The waiting time contributed to the whole effect too. It was extremely short.

The first thing this doctor told me was that he appreciated his colleague sending me to him and that he would be happy to help, but there was something he had to tell me first.

He was no longer supporting patients insured by the German Government.

In Germany there are two medical insurance plans, the Government Health Insurance System (GKV) and the Private Health Insurance (PKV).[17]

And this doctor was now only supporting privately insured patients, whereas I used the government system. Being so close to our move to Denmark, changing to another insurance scheme didn't make sense. Besides which, I didn't earn enough to be permitted to join the Private Health Insurance Plan.

So that meant that I had to pay to be treated by this doctor. He named the hourly price.

I said, "Please, help me. I will pay! I really need help because I don't know what else to do."

He nodded and said, "I practice both conventional and alternative medicine. Would you be open to an alternative, somewhat untraditional test?"

I eagerly said, "Yes."

He said that it was something to do with kinesiology. Now I know that this is "the study of the mechanics of

---

17

https://www.howtogermany.com/pages/healthinsurance.html

body movements."[18] But back then it was the first time I had heard the word.

He got me to lie on the examination table with my shoes off. Then he said that he would place various substances in powder form on my tongue, one after the other. After each one I had to push my foot against his arm as hard as I could. I would drink water after "tasting" each substance to wash away the effect of what I just had, and after a few seconds he would repeat the procedure with the next powder. If I remember properly, these powders didn't taste of anything distinctive. Only the texture seemed to differ.

It was the quirkiest and most curious test I'd ever done, and one of the most fun.

I did notice that the strength with which I pushed his arm varied from powder to powder, and even before we went through it all, the doctor said, "We have an answer here that can help."

After we finished I again sat on the chair adjacent to his table. The whole impression of the visit imprinted his office in my memory as one of the coziest doctors' offices I ever visited.

In my memory, he told me what I reacted to and created a nutrition plan for me on the same day. But the date on

---

[18] https://www.schoolofhealth.com/be-better/natural-health-definitions/kinesiology/

the nutrition plan says April 6, 2008. A month after the first visit.

I also found the results of many other tests and checks I had between the two visits. Allergy tests made by both specialist and privately owned laboratories, and those that could be performed for patients insured by the government. They showed that I had a slight grass and grains allergy (including wheat), a nut allergy, and one doctor mentioned dust. All of them extremely weak and almost negligible.

There was also something else among all those documents.

16. The Symptoms

That something was a questionnaire called Histamine Checklist, which I filled in during that month of intensive research and which tried to reveal what was wrong with me and why I was in so much discomfort.

I will tell you a little more about this A4-sheet of paper that lies next to my keyboard as I write this, and which I realize is extremely telling of how I felt then and of the chaos of symptoms I experienced.

But before that, just a few paragraphs on how great it is to find these old notes. It reminded me that the "alternative" doctor (as I think of the doctor today, to whom my physician sent me) suggested that I keep a diary of what I ate and how I felt after each meal.

I remember I made several attempts in my life to keep such diaries, both for my daughter and for me. When Emma was a toddler, we suspected she was having problems with gluten as well. I even bought a commercial version of such a diary for each of us, which I never completed. They both remained mostly empty.

I don't have that first diary or notes from 2008. At least I can't find it now. But this Histamine Checklist is a glimpse of what I was dealing with then.

The checklist was divided into three main parts.

The first one contained my name, birth-date, and the indication of my gender. Then I had to indicate how long I had experienced the symptoms and how often.

The "how often" part was easy to fill in. I chose the "very often (daily to twice a week)" clearly meaning daily.

I seemed to have had difficulty in recalling how long I had those symptoms. I chose the entry "1 to 5 years" but also made notes for "4 weeks to 6 months" and "since I can remember or at least for x years," which I amended to "at least 15 years." My additional notes stated, "strong," "acute," and "partial" for these three entries.

The second big part of the questionnaire had a list of thirteen groups of symptoms ranging from belly aches, nausea, diarrhea, and other indications of problems with digestion, skin problems, dry eyes, exhaustion, migraine, dizziness and possibly other. I had to indicate the frequency (with values "never," "rarely," "often," "very often," to choose from) and intensity ("weak," "medium," and "strong") of these symptoms. So, the frequency ranged from never to very often, and the intensity from weak to strong.

There wasn't a single symptom where I indicated "never" or "weak." Nine of thirteen were marked as happening very often, and six of thirteen being strong, with the rest being at least of medium intensity.

And the last part of the checklist was the list of the various types of food, listing drinks and meals, and leaving space for more entries of my own.

I marked most of them as being problematic and had only a handful marked with a question mark, not sure whether they were a problem or not. Besides, fruits, some vegetables (fresh and pickled), milk products, various drinks (both soft and alcoholic), various sauces including soy sauce, some types of processed meat and fish, baked products, I also indicated that I had problems with aspirin and mucus-relieving medication.

Finding this questionnaire now, as I write this book, reminded me of the chaos I was in then.

Besides that, I found the results of the asthma test I had half a year prior. I now recall how I fought with severe cold symptoms for many months in 2007 and 2008. But this additional document showed that I went to the lung doctor and complained of oppressed breathing for the past six months.

So, my physician had not only prescribed all the medication to relieve stomach aches, she had also sent me to other doctors to find the cause.

The most frustrating thing was that all those doctors were helpless and, in spite of all these symptoms, sent me home with the answer, "There's nothing wrong with you. You might feel bad, but the tests say your health is fine."

Today, I realize that in their place, I would be helpless too and shrug.

But at that time, I felt completely lost and abandoned to deal with my troubles alone. My situation seemed hopeless. What was wrong with me? Was I going crazy? Was I maybe, subconsciously, a hypochondriac making myself ill? Should I go to a psychiatrist instead?

As you can imagine, such thoughts were not fun at all.

P.S. That last thought reappeared when another physician in another country asked whether my multiple symptoms might be of psychological origin. Fortunately, at that time, I had other "data" on my symptoms, showing that something was going on with my metabolism, and my brain was not the only "guilty" one in the whole "mess" I was in.

[A side-note: Metabolism is defined as "the chemical processes that occur within a living organism in order to maintain life." — Lexico[19]]

---

[19] https://www.lexico.com/en/definition/metabolism

17. Nutrition Plan

So, the kinesiologic test I told you about a couple of chapters ago, was the game-changer.

Today, I am not sure whether this test and the tailored nutrition plan that the "alternative" doctor came up with happened on the same day. I previously believed this to be the case, but my records show differently. I believe he conducted the test on the first day we met, but I can't say for sure now. I contemplated asking this doctor for confirmation, but then, would it change or affect the story I am telling you now? No, it wouldn't.

It's worth repeating because it is important to me that you are aware of that. This book is not about finding each detail of my past to the letter, which is, of course, impossible. This book is about shedding light on how I moved from ill and suffering to hopeful; welcoming healing, and enjoying life many times a day.

What I clearly remember is how he explained what took place during that strange test. He said that he had me first taste something that all people are neutral to, to feel my normal strength. Then he gave the powders corresponding to various foods that are known to cause problems with digestion, cause allergies, or intolerances. He might have been the first to explain to me the difference between an allergy and an intolerance. The first shows a reaction independent of the amount of allergen, and the second gives a reaction only when a certain tolerable threshold is exceeded.

[A side-note: "A food intolerance is sometimes confused with or mislabeled as afood allergy. Food intolerances involve the digestive system. Food allergies involve the immune system. With a food allergy, even a microscopic amount of the food has the potential to lead to a serious or life-threatening reaction calledanaphylaxis." — AAAAI[20]]

He continued by saying that my strongest reactions were to gluten, milk, and fruit sugar.

After telling me what I had problems with, he suggested a nutrition plan. He sat at his computer and opened a file and shared with me that he had many patients struggling with food intolerances and sensitivities. To hear that was a big relief. I was not alone!

The file he opened turned out to be a template he had developed over the years, working with his patients and continuing his research in this area. It was a document, a little over five pages long, with many details on what to eat, how to prepare the meals (to cook or not to cook), and how to eat (how many times to chew each bit, whether it is recommended to read or watch TV during

---

[20] https://www.aaaai.org/conditions-and-treatments/conditions-dictionary/food-intolerance

meals or not, and so on). There was also a list of healthy fats and helpful food supplements.

Here are the last two lines of the document above the signature and a list of recommended reading, as I have interpreted them from the German. They reflect the whole tone of the document. I had never gotten anything like that from a doctor before.

"Exercise regularly, but not excessively. Enjoy the silence...

"Take care of yourself and: *EVERY DAY IS A BEAUTIFUL NEW DAY.*"

I have replicated the emphasis as it was done in the nutrition plan.

I still have the document. And even though what and how I eat has changed since I first read and applied it, this plan definitely changed my situation, my health, and my attitude towards it, considerably and for the better.

The plan was a reset diet, after which the doctor suggested that I try those problematic foods again, little by little, to see whether they still caused me problems.

The main changes in nutrition concerned gluten, milk products, and fruit sugar (fructose), but also some others.

In the later chapters, I will share how these changes altered my health and my life. Some more, some less.

My life didn't change immediately after I got my hands on this plan. And I still had some issues with my digestion and circulation. Less than a month after I got the new diet plan and started following a new diet, I had gastrointestinal endoscopy, and they found a type of gastritis and confirmed the possibility of food allergies. So, in addition to the new diet and several cookbooks and guidance books on gluten, lactose, and fructose intolerances, I purchased a cookbook with recipes for those who have irritable bowels.

18. Weight

I had tried diets before. The most notable was the Food Combining diet, which I tried out for my mom. She wanted to lose weight but couldn't. I discovered a little book on this diet, which I still have, and tried it out. I did lose quite a bit of gained weight. I eagerly shared it with my mom.

Neither my mom nor I stuck with this diet.

I guess it is easier to stick with a diet plan when your body urges you to do so, such as when you can't tolerate something and feel sick eating certain foods.

My weight changed considerably over the years. I was overweight as a baby, losing much weight while being a toddler, being very skinny as a teenager and young adult, and gaining a lot of weight in the first years I lived in Germany. Somewhere in the middle of the twelve years of my life in Germany, I tried the Food Combining diet. And although I didn't stick to the diet, my weight remained more or less stable until I had those huge problems with my stomach and digestion.

After changing to the gluten-free diet, I lost 22 kilograms (48.5 pounds) in just two months. That was scary for my loved ones, as well as for me. I was severely underweight and skinny again, my collar bones visibly protruding.

Then I started to slowly gain weight again.

During my first pregnancy I gained a little weight, but I lost it after the second. The second pregnancy took place after I had started practicing living in the moment and "being here." I realized that when I had bouts of hunger, I wasn't going to starve, since it wasn't long since I had last eaten. I started eating in small portions, felt much better, rarely had heartburn, and got a bit lighter again after giving birth to my daughter.

Just like my whole body, I didn't think of my weight too often, unless I felt reminded of it.

While in Moldova, many people reminded me to eat because I was so thin. Especially my mom. By the standards of those times, I was tall and skinny enough to be approached by a beauty queen hunter on a trolley bus in Moldova. I was already planning to or was attending my Ph.D. studies at the Academy of Sciences in Moldova at that time. So I said, "No, thank you."

I did think of this encounter a couple of times when I was overweight while living in Germany. I had no idea exactly why I had gained so much weight, and I will never know. Here is how I became aware that I was considerably overweight. I still smile thinking of it. I was even going to use this scene in my parable.

It was at a gas station in Germany. It was a trip somewhere with friends or one organized by the University Darmstadt, where I was working at the time. In the restroom was a high-tech (for those times) weight scale, like a slot machine. You needed to put in a coin, stand on the mark, and type a few data in. Now that I think of it, it was probably just one thing I had to enter — my height. I typed 172 cm and watched a small piece of paper that looked like a receipt being printed out. I expected to see my weight, height, and maybe also the price I paid for the service on that ticket. I didn't find those. They must have been printed on a separate ticket, which I either lost or disregarded because the one I held in my hand held my whole attention. It glared at me in big capital letters, "YOU ARE 13 KG OVER YOUR IDEAL WEIGHT!"

My mom had stopped telling me to eat more when I went back for a visit after being in Germany for one year. But this black-and-white statement in capital letters did scare me; however, not for very long.

I am glad that I didn't fret all of the time about my weight and my "problem zones."

Now that I am slightly underweight, while being on a self-tailored low carb diet, I don't think about my weight that often either. There were periods in my life when I fretted about my weight and checked it every single morning. They became rarer the kinder, the more honestly and more helpfully I treated myself.

I must admit that from time to time, I do observe myself judging how thin I look in some recent pictures, especially in those where I am not smiling. But I know that this "I am too thin" is not my truth; it is just a label I assign when comparing the way I look to the standard I set for myself at that point in my life. I also realize that these standards change, mirroring the changes in the opinions of our culture. Another possible reason is the fear that being a little underweight compared to a general norm isn't good, or might be judged as such. Once again, I try to fit in.

However distressing these thoughts and fears might appear, it is wonderful to become aware of these thought processes and not to judge them. When I look at my current state without judgment, I discover that I am doing well in terms of metabolism and that my weight has been stable (with only slight variations) for almost three years, since I started following a low carb diet.

So, I will trust life as it unfolds and my body to guide me to what is good for me, and if that means gaining weight, then I will gain weight and embrace it. And if not, then not.

And when I feel hungry, and stop resisting that hunger, I will go and eat.

Like now, for example.

See you in the next chapter.

19. Gameful Life

The previous nine chapters set out to be my backstory until now. You could also say that that was the actual memoir part. That part might not have sounded completely gameful. The reason for that might be that my gameful approach to life, and especially to my health conditions, is relatively recent.

Let me put this development into a brief timeframe. I started changing my diet and therefore moving towards the improvement of my metabolism in 2008. Until then, I had significant challenges with digestion, fatigue, dizziness, balance issues, runny nose, asthmatic symptoms, and others for many years, with the intensification of all of them, especially pain in the stomach, for a couple of years prior to 2008. At the end of 2011, I learned for the first time about the possibility of seeing myself, the world around me, and my thought processes non-judgmentally, in an anthropological way. In 2014, I was inspired to turn an activity into fun games. It was writing. In 2016, I started deliberately turning various projects and activities into games (and sharing this possibility with others, including the little book *5 Minute Perseverance Game* that I wrote and published that year) until, in the second half of 2017, I started turning all areas of my life into games. And I continue doing that today, continually adjusting my game plans to keep those activities enticing and fun, as well as to make progress with what I want and need to do.

The following chapters will contain some accounts of how I reacted to and handled various challenges in the past, but for the most part, they will reflect my view on them today.

And since I turn my whole life into fun games, my health challenges are no exception. Whenever I stop complaining about them and come back into the present moment of my life, I can become resourceful and approach them as if they were a game challenge.

And I approach them as both the designer *and* player of these games.

That is the best universal tool I ever tried out.

One of the most famous examples of gamifying (i.e., turning into games) big physical challenges is Jane McGonigal.

She is a game designer and one of the pioneers bringing game elements and a gameful attitude into real-life contexts. She was "the first to earn a Ph.D. studying the psychological strengths of games and how those strengths can translate to real-world problem solving," and used game thinking during her recovery from a severe concussion. As with many patients who've suffered a brain injury, she struggled with its consequences.

Then "thirty-four days after I hit my head — and I will never forget this moment — I said to myself, I am either going to kill myself, or I'm going to turn this into a game." — Jane McGonigal, *SuperBetter*

So she created a game, she later called SuperBetter, where she took on the secret identity of "Jane, the Concussion Slayer." Her sister and her husband became her allies. Everything she needed to avoid, such as bright light and crowded spaces, became bad guys, and anything that was helping her, like cuddling her dog or eating walnuts or going for a walk with her husband, were her power-ups.

[A side-note: A power-up is "(in a video game) a bonus which a player can collect and which gives their character an advantage such as more strength or firepower." — Lexico[21]]

In her acclaimed book *SuperBetter* also quoted above, Jane McGonigal wrote, "The game was that simple: adopt a secret identity, recruit allies, battle the bad guys, and activate power-ups. But even with a game so simple, within just a couple days of starting to play, that fog of depression and anxiety went away. It just vanished. It felt like a miracle to me. It wasn't a miracle cure for the headaches or the cognitive symptoms — they lasted more than a year, and it was the hardest year of my life by far. But even when I still had the symptoms, even while I was still in pain, I stopped suffering. I felt more

---

[21] https://www.lexico.com/definition/power-up

in control of my destiny. My friends and family knew exactly how to help and support me. And I started to see myself as a much stronger person."

After her recovery, she created a framework and an app with the same name SuperBetter[22]. Her approach has helped many people to overcome little and significant challenges and to do so in a much lighter and more gameful way than they would have managed otherwise.

I haven't used her approach, but instead created my own — which I adjust and re-design often as my interest and the focus of my curiosity change — while applying Self-Gamification.

Similarly to Jane McGonigal, I also stop suffering as soon as I play my games, whatever they are. That is whatever project or activity I perceive and approach as a fun game.

But how to enable that "end of suffering"? How can we be gameful? How can we live gameful lives?

Here is what Jane McGonigal says on that:

"To lead a more gameful life, you simply have to be open to learning about the psychology of games—and be willing to experiment with new ways of thinking and acting that can help you increase your natural resilience." — Jane McGonigal, *SuperBetter*

---

[22] https://janemcgonigal.com/ and https://www.superbetter.com/

I can full-heartedly back that up.

However, there is an amendment I would like to make at this point. You can be interested in and inspired by game design and game thinking, as well as turn anything you wish into fun games, *without* studying or researching game design or psychology in detail. All it takes is the skill-set enabled by Self-Gamification. By taking on the non-judgmental, one-small-step-at-a-time, and gameful attitude.

Here is another critical aspect when you turn your life into fun games. It is voluntary participation, which is one of the main parts of games, and in my opinion, the most important component for designing *and* playing Self-Motivational Games, that is when you practice Self-Gamification.

Here is what I mean by a Self-Motivational Game. It is a real-life project or activity that you adjust in such a way that it feels like a fun game with which you are eager and happy to engage, both in terms of its design *and* the playing of it.

I discovered that the most important component of a Self-Motivational Game, whatever it may be, is voluntary participation.

"Voluntary participation requires that everyone who is playing the game knowingly and willingly accepts the goal, the rules, and the feedback. Knowingness *establishes common ground* for multiple people to play together. And the freedom to enter or leave a game at will ensures that intentionally stressful and challenging work is experienced as *safe* and *pleasurable* activity." — Jane McGonigal, *Reality Is Broken*

I learned that in Self-Gamification, in other words, when I turn my life into games, the voluntary participation means the *will* to see my projects and activities as games, to design and never stop developing these games (that includes the will to learn from other game and gamification designers; also those who practice Self-Gamification and approach their lives gamefully), to play, which means actively engage in these Self-Motivational Games, and to have fun.

So for my health condition navigation games to be successful, I must be willing to see what I want or need to do there like games: design them, their goals, rules, feedback system, then test and play them, while following the rules I have outlined, and, through it all, be willing to have fun.

Please note, I don't mean that we should be expecting to have fun in the process. I discovered that it is easy to take suggestions from others and test out whether I like them or not, to prove it one way or the other. But what makes a game or any activity enjoyable is first and foremost, the willingness to have fun.

Thus, when dealing with health issues, I had a choice between despair (including the complaint, suffering, and so on) and being gameful (and through that also being curious, open-minded, resourceful, and trusting my heart and my gut).

But before I tell you about how I turned my health conditions into fun game challenges, we need to talk a little more about fun.

20. Fun

After exploring its various meanings while formulating and describing Self-Gamification, here is what I believe fun is. *Fun equals full, wholehearted, and rewarding engagement.*

Recently I started calling my daily life game "A Star Collector's Game," or "Ten-Star Game," if there were ten stars to collect. The number of stars varies as I adjust the design, trying out its variants. It is still in the design and test period, which my Self-Motivational Games hopefully will always be, because then they will be fun to "work" on, in other words, to develop and test further.

The element that I recently found myself modifying most often was how many stars I wanted to give myself, and for what.

This morning (shortly before writing this chapter), I experienced a lot of fun while doing a breathing and relaxing exercise that a friend suggested as a helpful challenge. This friend is, in addition to their day job, a Yoga and Thai-Chi teacher. He gave me the assignment when we went for a visit.

It would be adequate to say that it was my daughter visiting one of her best friends from kindergarten. She took her brother and us, her parents, along with her. Her best friend's family invited us for a pizza lunch, subsequent coffee for parents, and play for children. My daughter's friend has an elder brother who happens to be about my son's age so that each of our children had a play partner.

While the children were playing after lunch, we adults had coffee and tea. At some point in the conversation, I shared my latest adventure with osteoarthritis. I struggled with this health condition at that time, not able to look at it with a gameful attitude. In an attempt to help me, the father of my daughter's friend gave me the following fun challenge for two weeks.

He told me to do an exercise where I would stand on one spot and bounce my knees quickly, arms hanging down my sides, shoulders relaxed, and breathing deeply (in through the nose, out through the mouth). If I chose to and felt up to it, I could substitute bouncing with hopping swiftly on the same spot without moving the shoulders too much from their position. Then bounce again, then hop, then bounce, and so on. I had to do this bouncing-and-hopping exercise for five minutes twice a day, in the mornings (for example, after waking up) and in the evenings (before going to sleep).

His wife suggested adding, whenever I felt comfortable enough to do so, a variant of jumping jacks (star jumps) to extend my hopping and bouncing workout.

[A side-note: "A jumping jack (Canada & US) or star jump (UK and other Commonwealth nations), also called side-straddle hop in the US military, is a physical jumping exercise performed by jumping to a position with the legs spread wide and the hands touching overhead, sometimes in a clap, and then returning to a position with the feet together and the arms at the sides." — Wikipedia[23]]

Our hosts and I agreed to reconnect after two weeks and find out how I felt after completing this challenge.

Initially, I wasn't sure this quirky exercise would help, because bouncing my knees quickly while standing seemed too strange to me. I thought I would be imitating someone under an electrical current, and that for an entire five minutes.

But it did help. I felt much better immediately after trying it out, as soon as we got home. I also slept better that night. Since trying the exercise that evening, I haven't touched the painkillers for my joints. And before that, I was taking strong ones at least three times a day, sometimes more. These painkillers caused the unpleasant and disconcerting side effects of fogginess and a numb feeling in my head.

[Another side-note: The addition of jumping jacks (star jumps) to the bouncing workout increased my

---

[23] https://en.wikipedia.org/wiki/Jumping_jack

experience of fun and relaxed many muscle groups, especially in my shoulders.]

On the second or third day of doing this exercise twice a day, I started experiencing painful tension in my shoulder muscles, which I hadn't experienced before doing the exercise. Well, I wasn't moving that much in the past several months because many of my joints were aching, specifically my left shoulder. I kept movement to a minimum, which I am aware wasn't very healthy.

But on that day, even with the tension in my shoulders, I continued the hopping and the bouncing. Maybe because on that morning, I realized that the tension in my shoulders wasn't disturbing the fun I experienced during this quirky bouncing exercise. I just enjoyed noticing the pulling and pinching effect in my shoulder muscles while hopping, changing to bouncing, and then back to hopping.

I smiled broadly at the experience of fun, at the fact that I managed the exercise before bringing my children to school and kindergarten and starting my busy day. *Yes!* I thought. I collected all the stars I wanted to collect that morning in my daily Self-Motivational Games.

After that brief mental celebration, my "insatiable mind"[24] had a flash of an idea. *I could record a star (in my "Star Collector's Game") for each time I experience fun, then I will*

---

[24] I learned this brilliant expression from Ariel and Shya Kane.

know how many times I am aware of having fun, and maybe through this, I will be present, mindful, and aware more often.

But something was off with this idea. After the initial spark of the flash, enthusiasm disappeared.

I tried to work out why, but that only diminished my enjoyment of the bouncing.

So I let these speculative — and, I later recognized, manipulative — thoughts pass and concentrated on how my body and I (or the part of my brain that labels itself as "I") felt in it.

Then, about half an hour later, having accompanied my children to school and kindergarten, I understood what had happened.

The experience of fun in that moment had felt like finding a treasure. Then in the next moment, I could move on. But with the idea to record a star for each fun experience, I seemed to want to hold on to that experience for a bit longer, fearing that the next moment wouldn't contain any fun.

But trying to relive the fun encountered in the past would mean going back to the place where treasure had already been collected. I would find nothing there. The treasure would be gone, and there was no way I could discover the same treasure there again. I could look at and admire the pretty stones of pleasure I had already collected, but that newness, the excitement of first discovery, would be gone.

That was how I felt while trying to remember to record a point or a star for the fun I experienced, as well as fretting over whether I would recall the fun I had had doing whatever it was. I could see that, at that moment, all I could have felt was disappointment.

Just becoming aware of that was fantastic. Without planning to, I experienced fun again, by simply being curious about my thought processes, the world around me, and everything that was happening right there, right at that moment of my life.

That was when I realized the following.

Fun can only be found in this moment of life, and in being curious and open to finding the next treasure in almost everything.

Fun *is* the treasure we can find in any given space and circumstance, and at any given moment, regardless of whether the moment meets our preferences or not.

21. Gluten, the Mine

Gluten is "a mixture of two proteins present in cereal grains, especially wheat, which is responsible for the elastic texture of dough." — Lexico[25]

Of all the components of food, gluten turned out to cause the strongest symptoms in my body.

Just like for my fictional character Vivi, whom I mentioned early on, my stomach bloats considerably, and I need to loosen my bra so that I can breathe. My stomach also often reacts with a burning feeling. It seems to be different from "regular" heartburn because the burning feeling is directly in my stomach. However, the burning feeling is not the strongest symptom. The increased volume of my stomach is, along with the following.

A while after consuming gluten I will get dizzy and unsure on my feet. I have to support myself on furniture or ask someone to hook their arm under to support me until I reach something stable to hold on to, and then finally go to bed and rest.

I also become very pale, and when I talk, I have the feeling that I am speaking unclearly, although those who

---

[25] https://www.lexico.com/en/definition/gluten

listen to me usually don't confirm that. In all, I have to concentrate hard to formulate simple sentences, and I feel like I drank too much alcohol, feeling close to passing out, even if I am completely sober.

I also feel very cold and shaky. If there is a bed around, then I go to bed fully dressed and put on as many blankets as I can. If there is no bed or blanket around, then you will find me putting on almost everything I can find to warm up. Once when that happened at a customer's office after lunch, and the symptoms of my gluten intolerance hit, I put a woolen cardigan (which I sometimes carry with me just in case) over a sweater and a shirt I already had on. But that wasn't enough, so I had to put on my winter coat inside the heated office. And I was still shaking. So I had to have several hot drinks to warm me from inside. A couple of hours later, I could take the winter jacket off again.

In 2008, which was the first year after removing gluten from my diet, I tried testing bits of food with gluten deliberately after months of the diet to check if I could tolerate it. I couldn't. The last time I did such a deliberate test was Christmas time in 2008, where the Danish people eat those delicious "æbleskiver," which are dough balls fried in oil, and which you eat either with powdered sugar, jam, or both. Google Translate said that "æbleskiver" translates as "fritters" in English. Word-by-word "æbleskiver" means "apple slices," although, in their modern version, there is not even a trace of apple in the dough. But you could eat them with apple mousse, for example.

If you don't have problems with gluten and visit Denmark around December, I recommend that you try them. Although these days you can also find a gluten-free version.

So I tried one offered by my Danish teacher at the end of our lesson, enjoyed its taste immensely, but suffered as much the whole way home, which was about a twenty minute walk. I was afraid I would fall over somewhere on the street. But fortunately, I reached home and my bed without collapsing on the way. After that, I have never deliberately eaten anything that contains gluten.

Officially, I don't have a gluten intolerance, or at least neither German nor Danish doctors could find any hint of it.

Most patients that suffer from gluten get diagnosed with celiac disease, which is "an immune disease in which people can't eat gluten because it will damage their small intestine. If you have celiac disease and eat foods with gluten, your immune system responds by damaging the small intestine. " — MedlinePlus[26]

The gastrointestinal endoscopies I had, firstly in Germany at the beginning of 2008 and again at the end of 2008 in Denmark (after my husband and I moved to

---

[26] https://medlineplus.gov/celiacdisease.html

Aalborg in June 2008), as well as several thorough blood tests, showed no damage to my small intestine nor any considerable quantity of antibodies in my bloodstream.

But the symptoms were very significant, so all the doctors strongly recommended that I avoid gluten. And my body has thanked me for doing that.

Something else happened as well. Two years after I started following a gluten-free diet, I became pregnant with my first child. Before that, my husband and I had tried to create a family for six long years. After various attempts (including a failed round of IVF treatment and considering adopting a child), I became pregnant naturally with our son, Niklas, and he was born in October 2010.

Over the years, I was asked and wondered whether it was gluten, or a wheat allergy instead, since my symptoms were so reminiscent of a strong allergy, and so different from those of celiac disease. However, the same symptoms came also from consuming soy sauce and other products not containing wheat but containing gluten. Rye and other wheat-free but gluten-containing bread and other products had the same effect on me. So the observation with a scientific researcher's scrutiny led me to identify that gluten was indeed the issue.

Even in the tiniest amounts. One of the quirkiest stories I tell to illustrate this is when one evening, I felt sick with the "usual" gluten symptoms described above, although I had strictly followed the gluten-free diet. I was working from home that day, so I wasn't exposed to any possible contamination from an external dining place.

I adjusted my bra by hooking its extenders on the outermost pair of hooks, exhaled heavily, got a blanket, and started preparing to lie down on a couch in our living room while wondering out loud to my husband why I was feeling sick and what could have been the reason. We looked simultaneously down at our coffee table and saw the beer bottle. I hadn't drunk any of it, knowing too well that I couldn't tolerate it. But my husband had. He had taken a sip of it, and I had kissed him right after that. We were both dumbfounded. I knew that I was sensitive to small amounts of gluten, but that small?! This experiment has been unwittingly repeated, with the same results, several times since.

Nowadays, if I forget to check what drink my husband is having and I want to kiss him, if he points at his cheek I know that it is beer or another one containing gluten.

My symptoms come quite shortly after I consume anything with gluten. It starts with a burning feeling in my stomach, perhaps five or so minutes after. The full-blown effect becomes apparent at least fifteen minutes later.

What helps to relieve the pain and suffering is drinking a lot of water and sleeping for an hour or two. I am still tired after that but not as wobbly on my feet as I am shortly after ingesting gluten.

Gluten, and my reaction to it, have always been a puzzle for me. And not only to me.

Over the years, I have met many people with a gluten intolerance. I've met them either incidentally at a work meeting or social gathering, or through explicitly dedicated events put on by the local chapter of the Danish Celiac Disease Association[27].

Most of them experience the most common symptoms of celiac disease. Here is how the website Healthline lists them:

"9 Signs and Symptoms of Celiac Disease:

1. Diarrhea

2. Bloating

3. Gas

4. Fatigue

5. Weight Loss

6. Iron-Deficiency Anemia

7. Constipation

8. Depression

9. Itchy Rash." — Healthline[28]

---

[27] https://coeliaki.dk/

I have experienced some of these symptoms. I even had iron-deficiency anemia as a child. But while testing me for gluten, the doctors in Denmark detected that I had Alpha Thalassemia Minor. I will address thalassemia in a separate chapter. So the anemia could be attributed to thalassemia and not necessarily to my sensitivity to gluten. But of course, nobody could say for sure.

Many of my fellow gluten-intolerant folks, as well as doctors and nutrition specialists I have consulted over the years, are surprised at my swift and strong reaction toward gluten, and the dizziness and struggling to balance that I experience.

Two other people in my life have struggled with balance — my father and my daughter. I will touch on that topic along with its relation to gluten in the next chapter.

But for now, let's talk of something lighter. Here is how I associate my reaction to gluten, and what I need to do if I come in contact with it, with games.

The following game comes to mind. "*Minesweeper* is a single-player puzzle computer game. The objective of the game is to clear a rectangular board containing hidden 'mines' or bombs without detonating any of them, with help from clues about the number of neighboring mines in each field." — Wikipedia[29]

---

[28] https://www.healthline.com/nutrition/celiac-disease-symptoms#section8

[29]

I used to play *Minesweeper* quite often when I first discovered it. In the beginning, I just had fun playing it, but later on I used it as a means of escaping something else I wanted or needed to do. Just before writing about this analogy, I tried to play it again, and I felt the urge to come back to writing.

It never fails to amaze me when I see how turning my life into games has changed my perspective toward things I want or need to do. I now find the game of writing this book more fun than *Minesweeper*.

There might be times when I will enjoy playing *Minesweeper* again. But right now, it's just perfect as an analogy for my reaction to gluten. If I eat anything containing gluten, or figuratively speaking "step on a gluten mine," then I "explode," in other words, I stop functioning and have to "reset" my system (go to bed and rest) before I can start playing the game of avoiding the gluten "mines" again.

The clues to detect the location of the gluten "mines" can be as much fun to find and follow as those in *Minesweeper*, as long as I approach them in a gameful way. These clues for gluten are much more multi-dimensional than the numbers. These are the list of ingredients in the groceries we purchase, the menus and indication of allergens at restaurants and cafes, catalogs

---

https://en.wikipedia.org/wiki/Minesweeper_(video_game)

with lists of gluten-containing and gluten-free cosmetics, and other products listed by Celiac Disease Associations.

Sometimes I need to hunt for clues. I need to ask people for clues explicitly. It's a challenge. But aren't games fun because they pose challenges?

Yes, they are. I can choose to see reality in the same way, every step of the way. Every moment is a choice for the next step in my life's games.

22. Ataxia or Not

At least once in a while, many of us complain about not having enough information about something we want to know or have difficulties in understanding. But sometimes, once we get this new information, we wish we'd been left in the dark, because it opens a Pandora's box of even more questions, even more unanswerable than those before.

That happened to me with gluten.

I often wondered why my symptoms weren't consistent with celiac disease. I did read about gluten sensitivities that are not detectable through blood tests or gastrointestinal endoscopy, but solely through the strong symptoms of the patients. However, even in these cases, dizziness and problems with balance were rarely cited.

Then one day, I found it. And not only it, but even more things that had happened to me, which I hadn't previously connected with gluten intolerance. Such as the Bell's palsy in 2001.

I found this bit of information in an article of the German Celiac Society (Deutsche Zöliakiegesellschaft – DZG[30]). At the time I was a member of both the German and

---

[30] https://www.dzg-online.de/

Danish Associations and eagerly read their magazines containing new research, reports by fellow gluten-intolerants, and recipe ideas.

I was on a bus on the way to a meeting with a client. The trip took about two hours in total, around half an hour of which was spent on the bus from the main railway station in Aarhus to Lystrup, in the middle of Jutland. It was a cold winter day at the beginning of 2017.

I took the latest issue of the German Celiac Society magazine with me. On such commutes I usually take multiple reading options with me, primarily offered by the collection of books I have on my e-reader, with the addition of either a print out of an article, a paperback, or a magazine, as it was on that day.

At first, I was pleasantly surprised to discover an article that addressed gluten-related diseases other than celiac. There was a handful of these described. But I only remember one of these medical conditions clearly. Now, as I research for this book, I have tried to find the article in my collection of those I've kept about gluten and other intolerances, but I can't. I suspect I threw it away, because of the fears that appeared after reading it. I certainly remember having the urge to throw it away, but I can't say for sure whether I did indeed get rid of it, either intentionally or accidentally. It is possible that I saved it somewhere else that I can't recall today.

The fact is, I don't need the article anymore. Because if I search the name of this disease online, I will get references both for scientists researching the topic and laypersons interested in or affected by it.

You can tell that even three years after reading this article, I am still uneasy about the finding. More than five hundred words into this chapter I still haven't told you what the condition is.

OK, let me take a deep breath. … Here it comes. The name of this disease is Gluten Ataxia.

In the article I read, I first discovered the symptoms. These were dizziness, problems with balance, challenges with vision, unexplained Bell's palsy, problems with speech, posture, walking, running, issues with coordination, unsteadiness, problems with general movements, and fine motor abilities.

I was excited about finding many of the symptoms I had, which I could not find in the description of celiac disease and other gluten sensitivity conditions. But when I continued reading, my gladness disappeared.

I read a statement similar to this one:

"When somebody has gluten ataxia, the antibodies that are released when they digest gluten attack part of the brain called the cerebellum." — Medical News Today[31]

31

https://www.medicalnewstoday.com/articles/320730.php #what-happens-in-gluten-ataxia

[A side-note: "Ataxia is a neurological sign consisting of lack of voluntary coordination of muscle movements that can include gait abnormality, speech changes, and abnormalities in eye movements. Ataxia is a clinical manifestation indicating dysfunction of the parts of the nervous system that coordinate movement, such as the cerebellum." — Wikipedia[32] And: "Gait abnormality is a deviation from normal walking (gait)." — Wikipedia[33]]

In the article I read that day, I found that some of the doctors believed that if gluten ataxia was not treated, then it could result in cancer of the cerebellum, just like celiac disease can result in cancer of the intestine if untreated.

I gasped when I read it. My father died in 1983 from a stroke, shortly after surgery to remove the tumor from his cerebellum. I was ten years old at the time and can remember well several occasions when he fell due to balance problems while being fully conscious, and how distressing that was for him. He was an amazingly kind, optimistic, humorous, caring, and patient person. But his balance problems shortly before several erroneous diagnoses and finally the correct one about his tumor, were very painful and hard for him to cope with.

I was shocked. Did my father have gluten ataxia? Did I have this disease? I knew by then that I had the same genetic condition as he did in Alpha Thalassemia Minor.

---

[32] https://en.wikipedia.org/wiki/Ataxia
[33] https://en.wikipedia.org/wiki/Gait_abnormality

At least I strongly suspected that it was from him at that time, and later it was confirmed when my mom tested negative for it.

Was I also in danger of getting a tumor in my cerebellum at some point in my life, and suffering as he did?

Reading further helped me calm down a little. I read that not many doctors agreed that gluten could cause ataxia. But all who agreed also agreed strongly on one thing. The only treatment they saw as helpful was the following:

"Treatment is relatively simple and involves total removal of all gluten from a person's diet. All gluten, including trace amounts of it, need to be removed entirely from the diet. Even small amounts can cause the gluten ataxia's progression to continue." — Medical News Today[34]

By then, I was on the gluten-free diet and, most of the time, a strict one. From that point on, I also made sure to avoid all products with possible traces of gluten and stopped eating at markets or other places where contamination was possible.

After reading about the only possible treatment for gluten ataxia, I wondered whether my father might still

---

[34]

https://www.medicalnewstoday.com/articles/320730#treatment

have been alive, had he been on a gluten-free diet. But no one would be able to answer this question.

And whether I had it or not, the strict gluten-free diet was the right way to go, also testified by the lack of those strong symptoms of dizziness, difficulty with speech, feeling very cold, and bloated stomach, I experienced when coming in contact with gluten.

The calm didn't last long, although the fear for my life had been somewhat abated. Another fear rose in a strong wave washing over me.

Emma!

My daughter had issues with gluten when she was a little over a year old. It was the beginning of 2016, about a year before I read about gluten ataxia for the first time. Emma desperately wanted to walk, but she couldn't. She was falling often. We attributed it to normal walking trials without paying it too much attention. But then her daycare mom started calling me more and more often, asking me to collect Emma who was being whiny and constantly wanting to be carried. We were worried about this happening so often.

She wasn't ill, in a "traditional" sense, or at least, she didn't have a fever. Just an almost constantly runny nose, being whiny, and not wanting to be set on her play carpet or bed. I remember that I tried to connect her being whiny to the challenge of breathing through her nose. *Maybe it is just a persistent cold,* I thought. The cold was so much easier to cope with. I didn't dare think what else it could be.

And then one afternoon after picking her up early from daycare again, and giving her what I was also having, which was gluten-free, I noticed that she was in a better mood, more readily standing up, and more willing to leave my arms.

I consulted our physician, and she transferred my daughter to a children's clinic. Under the supervision of the doctor there, we started a gluten and lactose-free diet for my daughter.

The results were amazing. Within a week, Emma was walking. She was desperate to play football with her big brother prior but would fall after taking a few steps and become frustrated. Because of so much crawling, she even got cornea on her knees, which most of us have on the backs of our feet. But after a week of the gluten-free diet, she started dancing, keeping balance amazingly well, and climbing all she could. Her mood improved, she didn't want to be carried around anymore, and her cold symptoms receded considerably.

After about a month, we went to the children's clinic again. The doctor confirmed the improvement in her symptoms and suggested that we again give her food containing gluten. He explained that we needed to be sure that she had issues with gluten, and we might need to repeat this provocation several times before setting her on a long-term gluten-free diet.

The results of this gluten provocation were visible again in less than a week. My daughter stopped walking, became whiny again, and started searching for the support of furniture to move around. I called the doctor, and he invited us to come to the clinic again. Another month of the gluten-free diet and another relief of the symptoms ensued. We have repeated two more cycles of this. During the third time, I felt like I was poisoning my child, and I was glad when my husband took over and gave her bread. When I called the doctor after about a week again saying that her balance problems had returned, he called us for another consultation. His assistant observed Emma holding on while reaching for a toy and confirmed that she had deteriorated. It was determined that we should keep Emma on a gluten-free diet, and they also suggested we apply to our municipality for support with the higher expenses. We did so, and we were very grateful to get such support at that time.

The doctor at the clinic asked us to come again in about a year. We did so. Then he suggested that we start giving Emma milk again. She was reluctant at first, most probably because she drank rice milk instead of regular cow's milk while on the gluten-free diet and must have forgotten its taste. We started giving it to her with mash potatoes or crepe or inside other meals. In time she started consuming more milk products without any symptoms. And when I called the doctor at the children's clinic on the agreed day to report on Emma's condition, that she was doing well, the doctor said, "Start again with gluten."

I was worried, also because this suggestion came about six months after I had read about gluten ataxia. When I had that wave of worry about Emma, which I mentioned above, I relaxed again because, at the point of discovering gluten ataxia, Emma had been on a gluten-free diet for quite some time. So the only change I made then was to choose products for both of us without any traces of gluten.

But the suggestion by the pediatrician at the children's clinic to give her normal bread and other products containing gluten brought all those worries back. I expressed them to Emma's doctor, but he said that Emma didn't present like the ataxia patients that he treated. He said it made sense to try. Because, if Emma was able to tolerate those products, then it would be a shame to deprive her of eating as most other children did. Also, she was to leave daycare in a few months to join the kindergarten, where there were more children, and it would be harder to maintain a gluten-free diet. Although still worried, I agreed that it would be a pity to keep Emma on a restricted diet if it wasn't necessary to keep her healthy and comfortable.

So we started giving her normal bread, pasta, and other products containing gluten. Fortunately, she processed this food well and didn't have any problems with balance. She also maintained her great, merry mood most of the time, like she did during the gluten-free diet.

Of course, I was worried and watched closely every time she fell or crawled. But in those cases, it was just accidental and not repeated, or just a game. She easily stood back up, ran around, danced, and climbed.

So I relaxed and decided to trust that everything would go well.

However, recalling the article about gluten ataxia once in a while brought those worries up again. I had read before that problems with gluten could be hereditary, so my daughter could have inherited my issues with gluten. What worried me the most was that Emma, my father, and I, all three of us had, at some point in our lives, problems with balance, coordination, and dizziness. If gluten was a factor in causing these symptoms, wasn't I putting my daughter in danger by giving her meals with gluten?

But on the other hand, I had not actually been diagnosed with gluten ataxia yet. What if Emma had a protein problem, since gluten is a mixture of two proteins? My son had a milk-protein problem about a month after his birth. I experienced complications that meant I could no longer nurse him, and he had to have formula instead. Niklas got a skin rash from the products available in the supermarket, and the physician prescribed a special one from the pharmacy instead. Emma got the special product immediately after I stopped nursing, when the doctors and nurses at the hospital learned that Niklas had experienced issues with the milk protein.

I related this thought about the proteins to the doctor at the children's clinic in our latest phone call, and he confirmed that it might indeed be the case that Emma's symptoms were caused by protein malabsorption. This protein could have been gluten in Emma's case and the milk protein in my son's case.

Children grow out of challenges with problematic proteins, if they are given time without consuming them. And it did look like both of my children had managed theirs and were done with them.

At least, I hoped with all my heart that they were done with their challenges with food sensitivities and would never have them again. Practicing living in the moment with awareness and non-judgmental seeing helped me realize that even if I may wish so, I cannot control or know what will happen. Panicking or worrying won't help. So I can choose to relax and not burden either myself or others with occasional, fretting thoughts, and embrace my (or anyone else's) inability to know exactly why Emma felt bad eating gluten for the first year and a half of her life, only to eat it again another year and a half later and feel great.

Fortunately, I know that when strong symptoms begin you won't get cancer if you don't start a gluten-free diet immediately. I had the symptoms for several years, and now being on a gluten-free diet, my feeling of balance is restored, and I feel great today.

And, if my children ever feel similarly to me, they won't be in the dark as I was. There is so much more knowledge today than in the days when my father lived, or even when I first started the gluten-free diet, which was twenty-five years after his early death.

As I said in the dedication to this book, I hope that this account will help my children navigate any condition they might face. And I hope they will approach it gamefully. Not lightly and half-heartedly, but full-heartedly and being eager to be great, as in their favorite games.

While talking about games, let's conclude with another analogy between gluten and a game.

While thinking of how gluten "knocks me out" if I consume it, I thought of the Minesweeper I mentioned in the last chapter. Contemplating a bit further, I found another parallel. It was Ludo.

"Ludo (/'ljuːdoʊ/; from Latin ludo, meaning 'I play') is a strategy board game for two to four players, in which the players race their four tokens from start to finish according to the rolls of a single die. Like other cross and circle games, Ludo is derived from the Indian game Pachisi, but simpler. The game and its variations are popular in many countries and under various names." — Wikipedia[35]

---

[35] https://en.wikipedia.org/wiki/Ludo_(board_game)

I realized that if a gluten-token came into the same space that I (my token) occupied on the game field, then it knocked me (my figurine) out, and I had to "go home" and rest.

With the serious nature of my intolerance, and the possible effects of gluten on my health, I will always be immensely grateful for the presence of games, and both anthropology and kaizen, for inspiring me to approach my life in an aware, incremental, and gameful way. I don't know where I would be without it. Surely not in the good place I am today.

23. Milk, the Creeper

The strangest and, I must say, the funniest reaction I have is to milk.

If I consume milk products regularly, for example a little every day, be it milk itself or even naturally lactose-free products such as certain types of cheese, then at some point, I lose my voice. Completely.

Once I traveled to Finland for several days on a business trip. The hosts showed us a great restaurant that also offered gluten-free pizza. There, I ate one of the best gluten-free pizzas I'd ever had. I had it with a generous layer of cheese one evening. The next evening I was doing well, so when some of the participants of the seminar I took part in suggested we go to the same pizzeria again, I thought, *Maybe nothing will happen if I have another pizza tonight. The one last time was simply amazing.* So, even though I had experienced losing my voice from cheese and other milk products before, I thought maybe just two days in a row would be okay.

The day after the second pizza, I had to make a presentation for about an hour. It went well. My colleague, who was leading the seminar, took over. During his subsequent presentation, a question arose concerning the part I had presented.

I stood up to illustrate my answer on a flip-chart. In the middle of my answer, I lost my voice. From 100% to 0%. In the middle of a sentence. Or to be precise from 100% to 2 or 3%. I could still whisper audibly.

The man who had asked the question asked whether he had posed it wrong.

"No, no," I said. "It was cheese. I'm sorry!"

Immediately another question followed, accompanied by many chuckles and raised eyebrows, "Is our cheese in Finland so bad?"

I blushed and hurried to explain — in as loud a whisper as I could master — that the cheese was delicious, and the pizza too. It's just that I ate more than I should have.

Communication during the rest of the trip was much harder as I had to really force my voice in order to be heard.

More than once I have eaten too much of a milk product before a conference and had to make a presentation without my normal voice. Fortunately, I've always managed it, but today I try not to eat any milk products before a conference, or when recording a video for my online course.

Today my voice has also started to be affected if I eat too much of other things, such as nuts or seeds. These have historically caused a sore throat, while the complete and sudden loss of my voice has until now mainly been caused by milk products.

I'm still not sure whether it is due to lactose, which is "a sugar present in milk. It is a disaccharide containing glucose and galactose units." — Lexico[36]

Hard cheese, which usually doesn't contain lactose, affects my voice too, hence it is probably milk protein that affects me, rather than lactose.

Recent tests for various allergens, including food, were negative. So I don't know what it is. The fact is, my voice disappears if I drink a little milk or eat cheese or yogurt several days in a row.

So if you get annoyed by me talking too much, you might consider offering me a cup of milk. But please, don't ask me any questions afterwards. ;)

I just remembered something. I could tolerate most milk products without losing my voice while I was pregnant with both children. Drinking milk was still heavy for my stomach, but I could eat cheese and yogurt and enjoy other milk products every day. I love mozzarella, so I had it then. I hoped both times that this would remain after I gave birth to my children. But the loss of my voice reoccurred shortly after, which proved that my body gave my then unborn children and me a break, and then

---

[36] https://www.lexico.com/en/definition/lactose

returned to its normal — that is sensitive — state afterward.

Oh, and by the way, something similar happened with eating fruit when pregnant. No problems then, intolerant after. Well, what is there to do? (shrugging)

[A fun fact in a side-note: I craved strawberries while pregnant with my son, and apples with my daughter. The apples even seemed to reduce the occasional heartburn I had during my second pregnancy (with Emma). My midwife found it very strange since consumption of apples in large amounts typically causes rather than cures heartburn.

Another fun fact here is that my son loves strawberries. My daughter enjoys eating apples, but her passion for them is nothing compared to my sister's, who can eat an entire bowl in one go. Neither, however, compares to my affinity for them during my pregnancy with Emma, and even less so to Niklas' love of strawberries.]

So, which game character best represents my reaction to milk products? The Creepers from Minecraft.

"Creepers are a hostile mob in Minecraft. Possibly the most iconic mob of the Minecraft Universe, Creepers spawn in darkness, but unlike other mobs, they will not burn in sunlight. They silently move toward the player if close enough, and will ambush the player, giving off that short Sss...BOOM! And here we are, the Respawn screen." — IGN[37]

Where, "Mobs (short for mobile) are either passive, neutral or hostile." — IGN[38]

The creeper's behavior comes close to the effect that milk and milk products have on me. There is even this short "Sss" in the form of a scratchy feeling in my throat. And then, "BOOM!" The voice is gone.

---

[37] https://www.ign.com/wikis/minecraft/Creeper
[38] https://www.ign.com/wikis/minecraft/Mobs

24. Carbohydrate-Protein-Thalassemia Puzzle

Initially, I wanted to write three separate chapters on my problems with fruit sugar (and sugar in general), with carbohydrates and the condition that was discovered at the end of 2008, Alpha Thalassemia Minor.

The doctors in Denmark discovered it when I asked them to test me for gluten intolerance. The latter wasn't found, but the statement from the hospital after a thorough blood test indicated I had Alpha Thalassemia Minor.

I did a quick search and learned that "Thalassemia is a blood disorder passed down through families (inherited) in which the body makes an abnormal form or inadequate amount of hemoglobin. Hemoglobin is the protein in red blood cells that carries oxygen. The disorder results in large numbers of red blood cells being destroyed, which leads to anemia." — MedlinePlus[39]

So, it most likely explained the anemia I had as a child, as well as my slightly lower blood count and low blood pressure. I remember how, shortly after I got diagnosed with anemia, my mom bought black caviar just for me to

---

[39] https://medlineplus.gov/ency/article/000587.htm

eat to increase my hemoglobin values. She also made a mixture of lemon, walnuts, and honey, which I didn't like at first due to its strong sweet and sour taste, but learned to love in due course. I detested caviar too because my mom and sister wouldn't dare to eat it since it was expensive, and it was bought as a medicine for me. Now, no one would buy expensive black caviar for me. Maybe because my blood values have improved. :D

As I continued my brief research into thalassemia, I learned that there are two types of thalassemia minor. I was diagnosed with alpha thalassemia minor. Hemoglobin contains two proteins: alpha and beta, and I have issues with the alpha one.

"Alpha thalassemias occur most often in people from Southeast Asia, the Middle East, China, and in those of African descent. Beta thalassemias occur most often in people of Mediterranean origin. To a lesser extent, Chinese, other Asians, and African Americans can be affected." — MedlinePlus[40]

My father's last name is Ichizli, which is of Turkish origin, and as I learned, Ikiz means "a twin" in Turkish (Ichizli is the Romanian spelling of the name pronounced "Ikizli"). My father was made an orphan in World War II and was unable to be reunited with his family or relatives during his lifetime, but he did remember this last name and the first names of several family members. He also had memories of how goat

---

[40] See the previous footnote.

cheese was made when he was small, and that was characteristic of Gagauzia[41], an area populated by those whose ancestors came to Moldova from the Ottoman Empire.

I was almost glad to discover this disease, as a proven connection to my father. Of course, I already knew I was his daughter, and I have several physical features testifying to that, especially my eyes, my complexion, and my height (exactly his). However, discovering thalassemia and that it came from him was like carrying a bit of him close to my heart. The saying "his blood flowed through my veins" became even more literal for me.

Nowadays, many different services specialize in identifying our genetic inheritance. I might turn to one someday to learn more, and to find out whether I am genetically related to people carrying Ikizli, Ichizli, Iquizli, or other forms of this name and, if so, where we are all placed in our genetic family tree. Going in that direction might also bring more understanding to my health conditions. I see a real possibility for me to do that. However, that would be a topic for a different book. A person's journey is a whole colorful library, and the book you are reading now is about finding a gameful way to approach my health conditions and continuous healing. No more, no less. Thus, let's go back to what I discovered during my online research.

------

[41] https://en.wikipedia.org/wiki/Gagauzia

With all the discoveries described above, and which I had already made by the end of 2008, I still hadn't ever researched whether there was a connection between thalassemia and food intolerances. Writing this book finally nudged me into doing so. Very quickly, I found a few resources.

Here is what else came up upon conducting this recent research — I discovered that other people with thalassemia also have issues with gluten, and not just with that, but also carbohydrates in general. Especially those I call "natural carbohydrates," the products that have a high percentage of carbohydrates in their raw/original state, such as potatoes, rice, corn, wheat, and so on.

About three years ago, I went to my physician because I was feeling constantly exhausted and unwell again. The challenges with digestion, fatigue, stomach ache, and other symptoms had returned. She suggested that I eat vegetables.

"But they make me bloat," I protested.

"Well," she said, "bloating doesn't seem to me to be as problematic a symptom as the others you described."

I nodded reluctantly, but I still resisted her advice. Instead I continued trying a number of new gluten-free products, such as quinoa, which had become more and more popular.

[A side-note: "Quinoa is a grain crop that is grown for its edible seeds. It's pronounced KEEN-wah. It technically isn't a cereal grain, but a pseudo-cereal. In other words, it is a seed, which is prepared and eaten similarly to a grain. Quinoa was an important crop for the Inca Empire. They referred to it as the "mother of all grains" and believed it to be sacred. It has been eaten for thousands of years in South America and only recently became a trend food, even reaching superfood status." — Healthline[42]. Superfood is "A nutrient-rich food considered to be especially beneficial for health and well-being." — Lexico[43]]

On one evening at our house when my niece and her then-boyfriend, now husband, were visiting, I complained about unease in my stomach, although all I had eaten was a salad that contained quinoa. "Yeah," my niece said, nodding, "Quinoa contains a lot of carbs."

That stopped me. On the advice of her doctors, my niece was on a low-carb, high-fat diet, and had been for quite some time.

Hmm, I thought. I said that I wanted to try out the diet my niece was following and asked her for details. That was the first evening I started systematically following a low-carb diet.

---

[42] https://www.healthline.com/nutrition/11-proven-benefits-of-quinoa

[43] https://www.lexico.com/en/definition/superfood

Within a couple of days, something strange happened. The fog I hadn't really been aware of, left my brain, and I could think clearly. I was feeling less and less exhausted even on the days when I didn't have enough sleep.

I started to notice more often when I was satisfied and could stop eating. Before that, I thought I was constantly hungry. But that was just a painful feeling in my stomach, which I often mistook for hunger.

Now I can differentiate between true hunger and the "Wait, something in what you ate wasn't good for you!" message.

I started eating fresh salads for every meal and eating more vegetables than before, and rather than get worse, as I expected, the bloating receded.

As I started recovering more and more, I realized how one-sided my gluten-free diet had been for years. Almost all of the products I ate, even the chocolate cream, contained rice. Around the time that I started the low-carb diet, I discovered that rice proteins had a similar structure to both gluten and dairy products, such as milk and cheese, as well as corn, yeast, millet, and oats[44]. As a result some people's bodies mistook these other proteins with gluten and reacted in similar intolerant ways. It didn't mean that my body definitely did that too, but

---

[44] https://www.amymyersmd.com/2017/06/gluten-cross-reactivity/

reading about it as a possible explanation for my symptoms toward my gluten-free diet was very helpful.

It was amazing to see that I had blamed vegetables for years, only to discover that it wasn't them but carbohydrates that caused my overall exhaustion and sensitive stomach.

And then, while researching for this book, I found an article stating the following in summary: "β-thalassemia minor is characterized by reduced β-haemoglobin chain synthesis and sometimes mild anaemia, although carriers of β-thalassemia minor are usually clinically asymptomatic. Nonspecific abdominal complaints may be caused by gastrointestinal carbohydrate malabsorption (lactose and fructose) and/or malabsorption of biogenic amines (histamine), or proteins (gluten)." — Wolfgang J. Schnedl et al.[45]

Carbohydrate malabsorption?! And problems with protein, such as gluten?

Wow!

---

[45] Wolfgang J. Schnedl, Michael Schenk, Sonja Lackner, Sandra J. Holasek, and Harald Mangge, "β-thalassemia minor, carbohydrate malabsorption and histamine intolerance," — PMC (https://www.ncbi.nlm.nih.gov/pmc/articles/PMC563765 2/)

Then I found a blogger who wrote the following in her blog post about her life with thalassemia minor: "I know I don't respond very well to gluten. I can eat it, but after a certain number of times, there seems to be a turning point where I need to pay the price." — The Green Creator[46]

Only recently I thought I should give up on my wish of finding a single reason for my various food intolerances. But there might be one after all.

Finding this bit of information was like finding a crucial piece of a large, complex puzzle, needed to make the picture recognizable.

It might not be the last piece, but now my problems with a long list of products start to make sense.

The first key piece of the puzzle in understanding the situation was when I discovered low-carb diets, and experienced a positive effect on my health. As well as learning that crystalline sugars, fructose, and glucose are all carbohydrates. I was wondering why I had problems with them all in one way or another. Why didn't glucose help me much with my problems with fructose, as it did others who had fruit sugar intolerance? Both are "dietary monosaccharides, along withgalactose, that are absorbed directly into blood during digestion." — Wikipedia[47].

---

[46] https://thegreencreator.com/my-life-with-thalassemia-minor/

[47] https://en.wikipedia.org/wiki/Fructose

My body, I have now determined, will not accept too many sugars, be they simple (monosaccharides) or complex ones (as in rice and others).

Learning that there is a collective term, Gastrointestinal (GI) malabsorption, for various food intolerances was the major key to the puzzle.

"Gastrointestinal (GI) malabsorption is caused mainly by carbohydrates (lactose and fructose), biogenic amines (e.g., histamine), and proteins (gluten), and shows nonspecific abdominal symptoms." — Wolfgang J. Schnedl et al[48]

The authors of this article might never know the relief they brought to someone with these "nonspecific abdominal symptoms" and the "click" of a lock I heard opening when I learned that thalassemia minor and GI (I love how that acronym sounds!) malabsorption are connected. Even though the thalassemia minor described by the authors of this article refers to the beta rather than alpha version, I wasn't that wrong to draw a parallel between the patients the authors helped and myself.

The door of my "Food Intolerance Escape Room" was then opened completely when I read what had been done to relieve the symptoms of the patients with thalassemia minor: "In two patients with β-thalassemia minor we tested GI malabsorption, and diagnosed

---

[48] See the previous footnote for Wolfgang J. Schnedl et al.

carbohydrate and histamine malabsorption. Both patients with nonspecific abdominal complaints due to carbohydrate and histamine malabsorption recovered with an individual diet free of symptom triggering carbohydrates and histamine."

[A side-note: Escape Room is "a game in which participants confined to a room or other enclosed setting (such as a prison cell) are given a set amount of time to find a way to escape (as by discovering hidden clues and solving a series of riddles or puzzles)." — Merriam Webster[49]]

Well, it took me a couple of years of trial and error, but my specially tailored diet is now exactly that — it is free from "symptom triggering carbohydrates," as well as "symptom triggering" ingredients, such as nuts (and seeds), gluten, and dairy. And I do feel like I have recovered from most of the symptoms I had.

As I explore the world behind the door of my symptomatic "Escape Room," I also discover fun things about thalassemia, which I recognize in myself too:

"Funny fact is that many people with Thalassemia have a low heat tolerance and often feel cold (cold hands and feet). I personally don't like hot temperatures, since it makes me feel nervous/restless. So tanning in the sun is

---

[49] https://www.merriam-webster.com/dictionary/escape%20room

not something that I do or enjoy. I prefer a seat in the shade with my cold hands haha. " — The Green Creator[50]

---

[50] See the previous footnote for The Green Creator.

25. Going Nuts (and Seeds)

I was pondering how to gamefully title the chapter on nuts.

I have a slight nut and seeds allergy, the latter associated with my grass allergy.

They are so weak that when I eat just a few nuts or seeds, I feel quite well. And they perfectly complement a low-carb, high protein or fat diet. And they are tasty! Often, I end up eating more and more, until I have a hard time stopping.

I recalled how my mom-in-law ordered me to stop "inhaling" nuts during the Christmas holidays of 2018. The summer before I had eaten too many almonds and it caused my throat to become very sore. And that winter she saw me eating another type of nuts (I don't remember now which; it might have been a mixture of walnuts, cashews, pecans, peanuts, and probably also almonds and some others too) at an increasing rate. They call it "Heißhunger" in German (directly translated to "hot hunger"), which means "cravings." So she stopped me and reminded me that I feel sick after eating too many nuts. So I went "nuts" while eating nuts. And my mom-in-law (who I am lucky to name as one of my very best friends) was right.

Hence the title of this chapter, "Going Nuts (and Seeds)."

It does sound fun, but it has no connection to games. So I decided to Google "games with nuts." To my delight, I found that there is not just a board game called *Nuts!*[51] and a puzzle *Crazy Go Nuts*[52], but an entire board game publisher in France called "Nuts! Publishing"[53].

My cravings for nuts as soon as I eat a little bit of them could also be associated with the Cookie Monster[54] and his cravings for baked goods.

If I observe myself closely, kindly, and with interest, as an anthropologist would, along with the signals from my stomach, I can identify the threshold when I need to stop eating them. That feeling of, "Now, that's enough. A little more, and you will think you are hungry again." So basically, a red flag, a red card, and I need to clear the "nuts" field. If I ignore this red card or try to fool myself by consuming a small amount of nuts every day, without giving myself a longer break, then I will be disqualified, dismissed, and unable to play the "being healthy and feeling well in myself" game for at least some time.

P.S. Sometime after I sent the manuscript of this book to my editor, I accidentally discovered another game with the word "nuts" in the title. *Go Nuts For Donuts!*[55] is

---

[51] https://boardgamegeek.com/boardgame/96188/nuts

[52] https://www.miniclip.com/games/crazy-go-nuts-2/en/

[53] https://www.nutspublishing.com/eshop/index.php

[54] https://en.wikipedia.org/wiki/Cookie_Monster

described as "The Pastry-Picking Card Game." My children's favorite pastry is donuts, and they always ask for them when we write down our grocery list. The chocolate frosted ones are a particularly big hit. Soon after, I bought the game, and we all fell in love with it. I can't eat donuts because of all the intolerances I have, but this game — with its goal of collecting or getting rid of various types of donuts to obtain the most points at the end — inspired me to change some of the rewards in my Self-Motivational Games from stars to donuts. I can't eat donuts, but at least I can collect them! Besides which, donuts are easy to draw and color in.

---

[55] https://gamewright.com/product/go-nuts-for-donuts

26. Sorbitol Bug

Sorbitol, xylitol, and other "-tols" turned out to be something else I fooled myself with.

These "villains" I am talking about are sugar alcohols, which "can block the already malfunctioning transport system in the intestines of people affected by fructose malabsorption. These substances should thus be strictly avoided. Some of these substances are sorbitol (aka. glucitol) or mannitol (aka. Mannite, manna sugar). These substances tend to be used in chewing gum, sweets and ready meals. You can find the corresponding E-numbers in the ingredients dictionary. Xylitol and other sugar alcohols should also be avoided during the fructose restriced diet, but can be re-introduced in the test phase." — Food Intolerance Network[56]

[A side-note with more information: The E-Numbers used in the European Union: Sorbitol (E420), Mannitol (E421), Isomalt (E953), Maltitol, maltitol syrup (E965), and Xylitol (E967, xylite)." — Source: Food Intolerance Network[57]]

---

[56] https://www.food-intolerance-network.com/food-intolerances/fructose-malabsorption-intolerance/basic-facts-dietary-fructose-intolerance.html

[57] See the previous footnote.

Here is how I fooled myself. At the end of 2017, I was prescribed a strong antibiotic for periodontal disease, which brought with it some of the most severe side effects I've ever had. The treatment helped, but the dental hygienist at the practice (to which I had just recently moved), suggested that I rinse my mouth with a special solution proven to prevent periodontal disease. I asked her whether the solution contained sorbitol, since I had previously had issues when consuming it. We checked the ingredients list, and it did. After a few seconds of contemplation, I decided to try it anyway, thinking that maybe if I used the solution in the evenings, then the effect of sorbitol would have passed by the morning, and I wouldn't have any problems during the day.

The instructions for the solution was to rinse your mouth with it after brushing and flossing your teeth, without subsequent rinsing with water.

Well, it seemed to go well for the first few days. So I continued using it for some months. Then a strange cold appeared. No fever, but a runny nose, sneezing, and difficulty breathing through my nose. I also started having more and more problems with my meals. I started bloating, even while eating my normal salads with very low fructose content. This strange cold was worsening, and my digestion as well.

To my surprise, I stopped enjoying coffee. Espresso is my favorite drink, along with still water, and I was disappointed that it didn't taste as it did before. But I started tolerating tea again, so I bought many different blends of tea.

At first, I didn't connect the strange change to my sense of taste, my digestion, and the strange "cold" making my throat and mucous membrane very dry.

Then it hit me. *Oh my, it could be sorbitol!* Through not rinsing my mouth after using the solution, the sorbitol entered my system and reached my gut after every use. And by using the solution for so many months (if I am correct it was for at least half a year), even if only once a day instead of twice a day as recommended by the producers of this preventive solution, I collected sorbitol inside me most probably quicker than my body could get rid of it.

I had known for a very long time that sorbitol and other sugar alcohols weren't good for me. But I had hoped it wouldn't be so bad if I used it only once a day.

I decided to test my hypothesis and stopped using the solution. Within a few days, the symptoms started to ease up, and after a month, the strange "cold" disappeared. My digestion also recovered with time, and I could enjoy my usual green salads with meat or fish without bloating.

To my surprise, I discovered that I didn't need this remedy for my gums and teeth. The sorbitol-free toothpaste I am using maintains the natural color of my teeth, and my electric toothbrush plus flossing keeps my teeth clean and healthy. When I went for a check- up a couple of months later, the nurse said upon hearing that I'd stopped using the solution, "Whatever you are doing, continue doing it. It works very well, and there are no signs of periodontal disease."

When I tried to search for a game connected to the phrase "fooling myself," I only found the lyrics of a song by Eric Martin.

"Than the truth begins to hurt

It gets too hard to hide

I'm only fooling myself

I'm playing games with my heart and soul

"I know that fooling myself

Can be dangerous, dangerous

If I lose control

I'm only fooling myself"

— Eric Martin, "I'm Only Fooling Myself"[58]

58

https://www.lyrics.com/lyric/4306835/Eric+Martin/I%27m+Only+Fooling+Myself

If the sorbitol's effects on me were not necessarily dangerous, they were certainly extremely unpleasant. So it wasn't quite a "Creeper," but it was a "bug," which I planted myself.

I am glad that at some point I managed to "debug" my system of it, and gained experience for other possible cases.

27. Eyes and Foggy Vision

A website offering free online games[59] has the abbreviation FOG.

Well, I have another relationship with fog.

That is how my vision is right now for everything more than a couple of meters away.

I'm shortsighted. As per the most recent measurements taken by one of the many opticians I've had over the years, one eye has -2.5 and another -2.75 diopters.

But I can't wear glasses or contact lenses.

At the end of 2008 or sometime in 2009 (I can't remember exactly), I lost consciousness, fell, and my chin required several stitches. I felt dizzy for several days afterwards and thought that maybe my blood sugar was too low, having lost considerable weight on my gluten-free, milk-free, and low-sugar diet. But after some time trying to keep my blood sugar at normal values, I still felt strange on my feet, as well as having enormous migraine-like headaches. I called in sick at work. I took my glasses off and had a nap.

---

[59] https://www.freeonlinegames.com/

I got up and for some reason forgot to put my glasses back on. A couple of hours later, I realized I'd forgotten them, but as I was about to put them on it occurred to me that the headache was gone.

I reported this to my optician, and she suggested trying half-strength glasses, about minus one diopter each. That helped for some time, but I couldn't see very well at long distances.

I quit driving, as I'd get migraines with glasses but couldn't see well enough without them or with half-strength glasses.

I got stronger glasses again at a later point, and the migraines came back. The optician and I tried out various solutions. In addition to half and full strength glasses, I also tried some three-quarter strength and those with a smooth transition. The migraine would often start just five to ten minutes after wearing the glasses. Shortly before I stopped driving altogether, I remember driving for fifteen minutes or so before having to ask my husband to take over, the headaches were so strong and I couldn't concentrate on the road.

In 2017, I got my glasses changed three or four times. I also went to the eye doctor several times. At some point, he discovered that when focusing on one object and then moving to look at another object, my eyes didn't do so simultaneously. My right eye was slower than the left one.

The doctor gave me eye exercises. At first, I resisted doing them; then, after turning my life into games, it was easier to keep them up because I was getting points and later stars each time I did them.

These exercises were beneficial, but I was still having headaches from wearing glasses, so I stopped wearing them. However, the foggy vision still bothered me, so I kept asking for help.

My ophthalmologist listed my three options. First, I could force myself to wear glasses. I told him I had done that for several years until it had become so extreme that I was again feeling dizzy and close to fainting. This feeling disappeared when I didn't wear glasses.

Then he told me about the second option — contact lenses. And the third would be laser surgery. He didn't recommend surgery and said that contact lenses could dry out my eyes.

I didn't want surgery and glasses didn't work.

So I tried to wear contact lenses. And they worked. I guess they worked because my eyes weren't hindered by the fixed focus of glasses, and they could move independently with improved vision.

The contact lenses worked well until July 2019. Then my eyes became dark red and had such a burning feeling that my physician suggested that I get tested for allergies. She thought that I might have developed some cross-allergies.

[A side-note: "Cross-reactivity in allergic reactions occurs when the proteins in one substance (typically pollen) are similar to the proteins found in another substance (typically a food). For example, if you are allergic to birch tree pollen, you may also find that eating apples causes a reaction for you. Certain tree nuts also demonstrate cross-reactivity." — AAAAI[60]]

The blood tests my physician did were negative. Instead she asked, "Could it be your contact lenses?" I shrugged.

When I got the negative allergy test result, I decided to stop wearing contacts for a while. At first, my eyes felt unprotected and almost as though something was constantly cut into them. I looked closely in the mirror and saw imprints from the lenses on the cornea. That wasn't good. *That was scary!* An enhanced dose of eye gel and drops along with a good night's sleep slowly started to reduce the cutting sensation. After a couple of weeks, the redness was gone too.

After research online, I discovered that contact lenses could make the eye surface very dry. It was claimed that laser eye surgery could lead to even more dryness. Wikipedia names contact lenses and laser eye surgery along with allergies, pregnancy, and others as possible

---

[60] https://www.aaaai.org/conditions-and-treatments/conditions-dictionary/cross-reactivity

causes of "dry eye syndrome," which is "the condition of having dry eyes"[61].

I've had dry eyes for years. My mucous membrane and my skin in general are also very sensitive and dry. I use many moisturizing cremes, gels, drops, and sprays. Once a pharmacist at the pharmacy we frequented for many years recommended that I go and see the eye doctor after selling me many tubes of eye moisturizing gel. The eye doctor couldn't identify any eye disease, so he recommended eye drops in addition to the gel to use during the day.

Wearing contact lenses made the dryness of my eyes worse. And when I realized that, I also recalled my eye doctor warning me about the over-use of contacts, as well as a warning in the letter from the optician that accompanied the first package of lenses. They even offered a free pair of glasses for all customers who wore contact lenses, as a means of limiting their use.

I was so happy that I could see better with contact lenses, without the migraines, that I completely ignored these warnings.

Now, I am back to foggy vision.

But I haven't given up my gameful, and that means resourceful and fully engaged, approach to life. As the designer of my own Self-Motivational Games, I have

---

[61] https://en.wikipedia.org/wiki/Dry_eye_syndrome

adjusted my game plan to include taking care of my vision.

To assist the doctors in their search for a solution (the doctors at the local hospital have now taken on this challenge), I have added another challenge for myself.

Years ago in Moldova (it must have been 1997 or 1998), I got a quirky pair of glasses, Laser Vision. I was shortsighted then too, but after a check by an eye doctor who was a friend of a friend of my sister's, I was told that I wasn't shortsighted, that my eyes were just too tired and I should sleep more and wear these quirky black glasses with small holes in them for some time every day.

The producers and the vendors claim on their sites and in results of clinical tests[62] that "Laser Vision glasses can improve and even restore your eyesight."— INVET-ENART[63]

I tried to wear them, but I wasn't very disciplined either with sleeping more or wearing the glasses. So at some point, I got regular glasses when I lived in Germany.

But recently, after giving up glasses and contact lenses, I recalled the Laser Vision glasses again. After diligently wearing them for the recommended half an hour (this time split into six or three slots of five and ten minutes

---

[62] http://www.invet.net/laser-vision-clinical-reports.php

[63] http://enart.info/laser-vision-glasses/

each) for at least two months, I have noticed that I don't need to lean as far over our sink as before to see myself clearly in the mirror. So I might see slightly better than before.

[An update: The recent tests done after I finished writing this manuscript showed that the vision in my left eye has improved by almost one diopter, while my right eye has remained as it was.]

Also, outside, I don't feel as uncomfortable as I did. I am even able to recognize signs about departing times of public transport.

The adventure with my eyes is ongoing. And my recent check at the hospital was good fun. Except perhaps when I got the drops that widen (dilate) your pupils. The side effects weren't great, but writing longhand for this book helped to bridge time and to focus my attention on an activity I am passionate about. The remaining tests were curious and enjoyable, with all the movements for my eyes and three-dimensional pictures.

The doctors at the hospital in Aalborg want to see me again in a couple of months to find a solution that will enable me to see more clearly over distances without a migraine from wearing glasses. Their current guess is that the glasses I've had so far have overstimulated my eyes. In other words, the glasses were too strong, despite matching the measurements made during the eye exam.

[Another update: The medical personnel at the hospital recently tried me with some test glasses, taking into account the increased difference between the vision in each eye. After wearing these test glasses for half an hour, the excruciating migraine returned. So, glasses are still a no go for me. The specialists at the hospital in Aalborg are taking time to discuss the next steps in finding a solution for my eyes and vision. I'm looking forward to finding out what we will do next.]

It is quite tricky to pin this foggy adventure to a certain game. Maybe it is a labyrinth or another type of adventure, a virtual foggy world with many discoveries along the way. My life is full of surprises, all of them teaching me something new about myself and the world around me; so many colorful aspects to it, if I am there to fully appreciate them.

28. Perfume

My story with perfume turned out to be very similar, but maybe a little more "ancient", to the one with sorbitol.

I loved bragging about my sensitive nose. I wanted to have special abilities, like my father and sister, and I wanted something unique, shared by no one else in my family.

My father had incredible eyesight. Once, in Algeria, driving at night along a road with no streetlights, he stopped the car, got out, and disappeared into the darkness, returning with a black umbrella. My mom still wonders how he could have seen the black umbrella lying there, while driving past it. She often recalls this "incident" when thinking of my father's extraordinary eyesight. We used this umbrella for many years afterwards, including after returning from Algeria to Moldova.

[A side-story: As a child, I lived in Algeria for three years. My father was a guest-lecturer in the physics of semiconductors at Annaba University in Algeria between 1979 and 1982. He died scarcely half a year after our return to Moldova. Thus Africa, and especially Algeria, have a special place in my heart because most of my memories of my father — I was between 6 and 9 years old then — were gathered there.]

My sister has amazing hearing. This wasn't so agreeable to her students, whose whispers she could hear from the blackboard at the front to where they were sitting at the back of an auditorium accommodating a couple of hundred students. There is another anecdote, when my mom and I were talking about something we wanted to ask my sister, while waiting for her to get home from work. We were talking in our regular voices; the apartment door was closed and locked. We had changed the subject by the time my sister suddenly opened the door with her keys, entered, and answered our question from before. She said she had heard what we said several floors below us in the stairwell.

So, I was always proud to "own" the excellence of another sense — smell. I could recognize smells from several hundred meters away. My favorite memory was when my husband and I walked down the old streets of Taormina in Sicily and I said, "Oh, somebody is cooking tomato sauce, and it smells just like my mother used to do it back in Moldova when I was younger." Michael said he smelled nothing. Several blocks on he recognized the smell too, and further still we could tell which window it was coming from.

When I became an author myself, I realized that the sense of smell was a time machine. I recalled how entering an Indian restaurant once transported me back to my great-aunt's house, where I spent many school holidays. Yes, this time machine often transports us to our childhood and other long-past times and refreshes the memories.

The trouble started a couple of years ago when I decided I wanted some aroma in my life. I stopped using perfume many years ago because even the faintest use of it was making me very uncomfortable. But at some point I decided using perfume-free toiletries was boring. Since I couldn't use too many, I tried doing a "trade" with my nose. I used facial cremes with some perfume in them, but perfume-free ones for my body. But I tried to fool myself again. I decided to start using a shower gel with perfume. I would be washing it away, so surely the smell would wash away too. Or so I thought. I would have the flowery aroma to enjoy during the shower and could then get rid of it by rinsing. But I was wrong.

At the same time, the producer of my facial cremes changed the recipe so that it smelled differently to what I was used to. I started frantically buying and trying different brands. All failed. Then I got a cold, and this was when it all got out of hand. I again started having asthmatic symptoms. I went to the doctor, and the tests showed no asthma. I went again, and when she looked at me, she said, "You look very sick."

I protested, "But I don't have a fever. Could it be an allergy, maybe? Perfume allergy. I seem unable to stand any perfume lately and start coughing in restaurants and buses when surrounded by people wearing various perfumes."

The doctor told me that there is no perfume allergy. Perfume is an irritant, and some people tolerate it better, some less. *Oh no,* I thought. *Not another intolerance!* I feared that the doctor would say, "Try to avoid perfume."

And that was exactly what she said. She helpfully named where perfumes could be found, and I couldn't stop thinking of what we had and used in our household, *Oops, that one has perfume too. And the shower gel!*

But I still didn't want to believe that what I had was a common cold. "I've had this for three weeks now," I said out loud.

"Viruses can take as long as six weeks to pass."

Six weeks!

I went home very upset. I was convinced I had some allergy. I even bought a nasal anti-histamine spray and used it together with an asthma spray that my physician had prescribed just in case during the previous visit. I had to admit that the asthma spray didn't help, although I believed that in combination with the allergy spray, it would.

I tried to convince my physician that I was right, and she said, "All I can tell you is that perfume does not cause an allergy, so the anti-histamine spray shouldn't be helping you. I can't tell you, 'Go ahead and use it.' That is your decision. My recommendation is that you go and treat your cold without using either the asthma or allergy spray, and try to avoid perfume."

I felt overwhelmed. "How can I avoid perfume? It's everywhere! I could hardly breathe on a bus on the way here."

"You can start by avoiding using it yourself."

Yes, my upset was enormous, and I went home determined to test her "tip," as she said and to prove she was wrong. So I kept the asthma and allergy sprays close by but didn't use them. I also canceled the appointments I had in the upcoming days to avoid infecting other people with my virus, in case I had one.

And I stopped using the shower gels with fragrances. Plus, I went on buying facial, hand, and foot cremes without perfume. They were much easier to find than I imagined. The Danish pharmacy produces a whole line of fragrance-free cosmetics — even hair wax. I also found great natural and perfume-free products by other Danish companies, sold in health stores.

I had another appointment with my physician three weeks later. She'd said that we could continue investigating my asthma once my cold was gone, to obtain reliable results.

I went to this appointment and thanked my physician. I told her that she was right about the cold, and that I had recovered without the use of either spray. I also told her about my illusion with the shower gel and how removing perfume from my toiletries, and the use of non-fragrant washing and cleansing gels and soaps had helped tremendously. Although I still feel a little on edge walking through a perfumery department in a store, or sitting next to someone wearing strong perfume on a bus, I am not as out of breath as I was before. The doctor told me how she and people in her family were also sensitive to perfume and strong odors and fragrances, and how they had to change seats in church or other public places if someone near them was wearing any.

I was grateful for her telling me her story only after I had experienced the recovery myself. That way she wasn't imposing her experience on me and let me find out in my own way, but when I shared my story with her, she shared hers and let me know that I wasn't alone and even such "mighty" people as doctors can have the same human experiences as us "poor" patients.

What did this story teach me? Well, first of all, that even after all the inspiring stories I've had with doctors, even now, I have the tendency to resist what they say. Secondly, that I (or my mind) can still fool myself, even having practiced seeing myself non-judgmentally and living in the moment for many years. Being kind and honest with and helpful to myself is a lifestyle. But a lifestyle is not something we can maintain all the time. Sometimes we deviate from the path we want to pursue. *A lifestyle is something we come back to as soon as we notice ourselves going off track.*

Becoming aware of this truth reminded me of one of many great quotes by my favorite authors about living in the moment, Ariel and Shya Kane, who wrote once on social media, "At times you will live in the moment. Other times you will repeat old behaviors from the past. Expect it and don't judge it!"

Thus basically, I, or rather my clever brain, at least once in a while — and probably more often — attempt to fool myself, as one wants to fool others in the game Mia or other Liar's games.

"Mia is a simple dice game with a strong emphasis on bluffing and detecting bluff related to Liar's dice." — Wikipedia[64]

"Liar's dice is a class of dice games for two or more players requiring the ability to deceive and to detect an opponent's deception." — Wikipedia[65]

Well then, let's play!

---

[64] https://en.wikipedia.org/wiki/Mia_(game)
[65] https://en.wikipedia.org/wiki/Liar%27s_dice

29. Arthritic "Rubik's Twist"

I mentioned my osteoarthritis several times in this book already. In the introduction, I called it "my latest adventure." And when I don't complain about it, it certainly becomes an adventure.

It might sound like it came on suddenly. But in truth, it didn't, and such a disease can't appear all at once. The pain in my joints was there for quite some time, but I ignored it until recently.

Well, I've had pain in the joints of my right wrist for many years now. But I blamed it on an occupation. I used to create Christmas decorations by safety pinning sequins into Styrofoam of various shapes. After learning that repetitive movements over long periods can cause chronic wrist pain, like the workers turning Champagne bottles by hand[66], I had the guilty suspect. It wasn't a person, but it was an occupation I blamed, and myself

---

[66] See 2.5.1.6 Ergonomic Hazards in "Introduction to Wine Laboratory Practices and Procedures" by Jean L. Jacobson, https://www.tau.ac.il/~chemlaba/Files/jean-l-jacobson-introduction-to-wine-laboratory-practices-and-procedures.pdf. See also an image of this laborious activity here: https://commons.wikimedia.org/wiki/File:Champagne-Remuer.jpg

along with it. I might even have blamed who or whatever had given me the idea for such a hobby in the first place.

I went to the doctor, and she recommended getting a more comfortable computer mouse, and resting the wrist as much as I could. I did both, and it helped.

But I still can't use my right hand as much as I did in the past, and also less than my left hand. I will often move a heavier object from right to left hand, or whenever possible, use both hands or my shoulders to carry such objects. Even holding one of my children's hands during a walk can become tiring after a while, so they kindly switch sides with me when I ask. Building LEGO for longer stretches, which for me means just ten minutes or even less, can also cause pain in my right wrist. So I stop building and search for the parts instead, and my children continue to build.

In June 2018 I had a hard fall on my left knee and chin, and both required stitches. A couple of months later I went to our physician, complaining about the pain in my knee. She told me that nothing was broken and no surgery could be done in such cases. I asked her if I could do sports. She said that I should decide about that and suggested I do it if I wasn't in pain and stop when the pain appeared.

Then about nine months later, I noticed a sharp pain in both of my knee-joints during a workout. I ignored it and pushed through. With time I was less and less motivated to do my daily workout mixed with Yoga exercises. Even if I included it in my daily games and rewarded with myself with points and stars, I was working out less and less.

Only when the discomfort in my left shoulder, which I had felt for many months, turned into a sharp pain, did I stop, and look attentively and non-judgmentally at what was happening. I acknowledged that quite a few of my joints had been aching for quite some time. Some less, some more. I suddenly remembered the nights when I woke with a burning feeling in my knees. Or how I took paracetamol because I felt like I had flu for days, my joints hurting, but with no other symptoms.

And when my mom told me that she had been diagnosed with osteoarthritis since before I was born, I realized how ignorant I had been, not only to my pain but to hers as well. I had acknowledged her pain before and even translated her symptoms to the doctor here in Denmark when I accompanied her to regular checks and consultations, but somehow, I forgot that she had struggled with this condition for so many years.

Writing this book also turned out to be an absolute blessing in this regard. I'm not only looking more honestly at what is happening and how I treat myself, I'm also purposely researching and learning from others. Just like a game designer eagerly tries the games of their peers and learns from them. So I started reading books by those who suffer from chronic pain. And here is one of the eye-opening quotes I found in one of them:

"Do not ignore your body's pleas to say no to an activity." — Toni Bernhard, *How to Live Well with Chronic Pain and Illness*

This sentence is written in bold as the title of a section in a chapter of Toni Bernhard's book. I love reading every word in the books I enjoy. But here I noticed I had an urge to skip the section. I noticed how I tried to hurry up. At first, I didn't know what that meant, so I stopped and went to do something else. That something else might have been reading another book. I don't recall exactly.

A bit later, I came back to reading this section and was able to look non-judgmentally at this discomfort. I saw that with all the pain I have been experiencing my body was pleading me to stop doing some of the exercises. For example, an exercise where I had to move my legs sideways and push through discomfort resulted in sharp pain, and stiffness of the corresponding hip joint the following day. I ignored all that, attributing the pain to muscle ache and not being fit enough, plus laziness, until eventually I stopped working out completely for several months, which didn't help either. I still got the sharp pain in my shoulder.

Yes, here came the lesson again: Do not ignore your body. Listen to it and trust its signals.

Maybe you will recall the story of me losing my voice when I consumed milk products. I only lost my voice if I continued eating these products for several days in a row. If I ate it once and then didn't for a week or so, then my voice remained at its normal level. In other words, it was only when I stepped over a certain threshold without "listening" to the slight tingling in my throat and feeling of heaviness in my stomach, ignoring the many signs my body provided me with, until they became so strong that I couldn't possibly ignore them anymore. There is no way to ignore losing your voice!

The same was true of osteoarthritis. First one joint hurt, then another. Then more. Is it bad that I was so ignorant?

Earlier I would have said "yes." Now, having given it some thought and thanks to my experience with Self-Gamification, I realize that it's not. Whatever we are up to or whatever happens in our lives, we treat those things in only two ways: we either escape from them, or escape to them while escaping others.

I ignored my joints for some time. But they called for my attention, so now I'm learning how to take care of them and my body. That is all part of learning how to be kind and honest to myself, as well as caring.

Because this is where kindness, honesty and caring for others starts — with ourselves.

While writing this book, I found this same idea in Toni Bernhard's *How to Live Well with Chronic Pain and Illness*. She describes how she applied a pearl of wisdom to relationships not only with those around her but also with herself. This wisdom was the famous "Buddha's teachings on skillful speech; he said that we should speak only when what we have to say is true, kind, and helpful." — Toni Bernhard, *How to Live Well with Chronic Pain and Illness*

I told you in the chapter about fun how I stopped taking painkillers. The friend who gave me the breathing and bouncing plus hopping exercise compared painkillers to the following scenario. He said taking painkillers is not like extinguishing the fire; it is more like turning off the smoke detectors.

That was quite enlightening to me. And even if my brain doubted what effect this quirky exercise would have on my joints and general physical state, I said "yes" to the challenge. Now, many weeks past the agreed duration of the assignment, I'm still doing the exercise in the morning and evening, and recently also a couple of times during the day, for five minutes each. I do feel rejuvenated and helped.

This exercise amazes me in many ways: its simplicity, the fun I have while doing it, and its fantastic effects. Both on my physical and emotional state.

It even feels like practicing meditation. I believe it is the closest I have come to a meditative state. I close my eyes during some stretches of bouncing, hopping, and breathing, and relax, observe what is happening in my mind and body, open my eyes, check the timer to see how much of the five minutes I have left, observe how the time that passed felt for me (short or long), which is telling of whether my mind is as relaxed as my body or whether I am in a hurry to get somewhere, close my eyes again, and enjoy all the moments of the remaining minutes. It's fun to observe my thoughts during those five minutes while bouncing and hopping interchangeably on the spot, all accompanied by deep breathing. There is a lot of space for all kinds of thoughts within five minutes. Many of them hilarious when not taken personally. And some of them also enlightening.

I sometimes play a game with myself, trying to remain on the same spot while hopping with closed eyes. It is fun to discover which wall in the room I am facing and where the new spot is when I open my eyes. Sometimes I manage to remain on the same spot, sometimes not. Once, before opening my eyes, I thought that I was on the same spot, then I opened them and found I was only a few centimeters away from hitting an open door, which was over a meter away when I started the exercise. I must have been hopping too energetically.

Also, in the physical sense, the results have been amazing. The more I practice this exercise, the fewer cramps I get in my feet and legs, even if I haven't further increased my magnesium intake. I am less often cold than I was before, and feel energized and merry after completing them.

In addition to the bouncing and hopping exercises, I also do some yoga and pilates exercises once in a while, and I've started dancing around the house. I read that the patients who danced and practiced aerobics experienced considerably more pain-relief than before. "In a study published in the 2014 issue of Geriatric Nursing, older adults who took a 45-minute dance therapy class twice a week reported less knee and hip pain and were able to walk faster after three months." — Arthritis Foundation[67]

So I dance more often and happily declare to my family that now I must dance. Also, I think of and treat each household chore as an exercise more often nowadays. I've tried to do so in the past, but today, when just standing up from a chair is difficult, and I can feel the joints of my fingers while typing, I am increasingly aware of any movements that *don't* hurt. I used to take them for granted before.

[An important update: While working on this book, I started reading *Eat Move Sleep* by Tom Rath. He has to deal with a severe chronic condition and embarked on an adventure to do profound research on what is beneficial for our health. He discovered and shows in his book that it is a combination of healthy nutrition, enough movement, and sufficient sleep.

Tom Rath emphasizes that sitting for long periods at a time might be detrimental to our health. "If you sit for hours on end, your blood sugar and insulin levels will spike to dangerous levels." He refers to "experimental settings," showing that "even two minutes of leisurely

---

[67] http://blog.arthritis.org/living-with-arthritis/dance-therapy-joint-pain/

walking every 20 minutes was enough to stabilize blood sugar levels" for those who participated in the studies.

He says that standing up can help, but "standing still for extended periods can cause unnecessary strain if you don't move around or alternate with sitting."

I can confirm that. Both sitting and standing on one spot while working at my computer for extended periods resulted in strain in my shoulders and neck, as well as intense headaches.

I found the following bit in his book curious:

"Working on this book was an experiment in itself. I decided to build a workstation on my treadmill and set a goal of writing this entire book while walking. So I mounted my computer monitor above my treadmill and built a homemade keyboard tray across the arm rests. Because it was a low-cost solution, I figured it was worth trying even if it did not work out.

"After using this homemade walking desk for several months, I am now walking *an additional 5–10 miles per day* as a result. At the end of each 'walk day,' as I have started to call it, my back no longer aches. I also have dramatically more energy compared with days when I am sitting in meetings, cars, or airplanes." — Tom Rath, *Eat Move Sleep*

I found that utterly inspiring and fun. So, nowadays I spend much less time sitting — often for less than two hours a day, and no more than twenty or twenty-five minutes at a time. I frequently walk around our house when I work on my books and articles, especially while revising my manuscripts. I read while walking, stop at different spots to make notes on the edits I want to make and continue the reading and walking. Right now, I am walking on one spot at my computer as I type these words. Every time I manage to sit for under twenty-five minutes at a time, I give myself a point, and at the end of the day both for short sitting periods and for standing, I get a donut. I call them "sitting" and "standing" donuts. It's silly and, therefore, fun.]

I'm thrilled that I haven't taken even light painkillers for my joints ever since talking to my daughter's friend's parents. I still experience discomfort and pain in my joints (especially in my left shoulder), but not as bad as before, and I am hugely grateful for that.

Discovering that I can experiment with various types of movements and find out which are not only pain-reducing but also fun for me, was great and reassuring. Here is an experiment I performed recently. Many recommend walking at least ten thousand steps a day. So I measured how many steps I was doing during my bouncing-hopping exercise. It turned out that I do about five hundred steps when I bounce and hop for five minutes. That would mean that I would need to bounce twenty times in one day to reach ten thousand steps with my current favorite form of workout. This equals one hundred minutes of bouncing and hopping every day.

Quite daunting! But if I adjust the design of my Self-Motivational Games by dividing the distance between the two or three of these exercises and twenty into separate levels, for which I reward myself with various types of stars or badges, then the whole process of leveling up ceases to look scary but instead becomes enticing and fun. (I'm happy to report that I got a couple of bonus stars for more hopping and bouncing since this update of my game design.)

[An addition to the update in this chapter above: The less time I spend sitting, and the more I combine it with standing and walking, the more improvement I feel in my posture and the strengthening of various groups of muscles in my back, hips, and legs. The pain in my hip joints recedes as well. So, walking while working on my books, which I love doing so much, removed the need to bounce for one hundred minutes a day. But I want to try to hop and bounce more. On some days, when I bounce and hop only once for five minutes, I notice that it is not enough. My joints tell me so, and more than once. So, I am actively trialling various game design elements to entice me to bounce more, as well as do more exercises for my eyes.]

A little earlier, while trying to move my leg sideways and experiencing a painful tug in my left hip joint, I thought of a great gameful analogy for my osteoarthritis.

Certain movements occur without problem, such as moving my arms and legs straight in front of me and up or down, but not all of the sideways movements work. It reminded me of a toy I loved as a teenager, and because of that bought one for my daughter, and recently a set of mini versions of it for my son's birthday party, for all his guests, him, and his sister, to play.

This toy is the *Rubik's Twist*, sometimes also called *Rubik's Snake*. "The Rubik's Twist is a toy with 24 wedges identically shaped like prisms. The wedges are connected, by spring bolts, such that they can be twisted, but not separated. Through this twisting, the Rubik's Snake can attain positions including a straight line, a ball, a dog, a duck, a rectangle, a snake, and many more imaginative shapes and figures" — Rubiks[68]

The specific triangular-rectangular shape of the wedges dictates only specific movements while twisting the toy. If you apply too much pressure, the plastic prisms break, as happened to the first *Rubik's Twist* I bought for my daughter. My joints behave in a similar manner. If I turn them according to their shape and current "abilities," then the movements are smooth, and I feel well, but if I try to twist them in the wrong direction then I am struck with a sharp pain. Shifting the weight and moving along another more suitable axis is the best solution both for the *Rubik's Twist* and for me to function and not break.

Somehow I love the idea that my joints function in a similar way to one of my all-time favorite toys.

---

[68] https://www.rubiks.com/en-eu/rubik-s-twist-1.html

30. The Daily Games

The previous chapters reveal my journey with health conditions so far. Some of the adventures are from long ago and some recent. Some have been told right after they were experienced, others remembered and viewed through a prism of collected experiences and lessons learned. But they all now lie in the past as I am finishing this book.

My future is unknown and not worth guessing (why spoil the surprise?). It will reveal itself moment by moment, one step at a time.

Thus, one question remains: What do my days look and feel like today?

Are they full of "Ouch! Damn. Not again" and "I shouldn't have eaten that"?

Sometimes. But not as much as before, and not with the same intensity and drama as in the past.

Turning my life into games affected and improved everything.

But what about this book? It is a game too. And this game is about to end. It all started with an idea for a novel, followed by the idea of writing a parable.

As you probably noticed, it didn't become a parable. I didn't write about the fictitious character Viviana, Vivi, and her mentor Jen, inspired by my dear friend Jennifer Nekuda.

Neither did I pursue the predecessor romance about Vivi and the handsome Italian heir of a pizzeria, Luca. Even though I already planned what the happy end for them would be. Luca was going to offer Vivi marriage and tell her that thanks to her, he discovered what he wanted to do in the culinary business. Before meeting Vivi, he thought he could either join his mother in a pizzeria or his brother in an espresso cafe. He wasn't drawn to either, although he was helping out with both, and didn't know exactly what he wanted to do. Meeting Vivi and learning about her challenges made him aware of people who had issues not only with gluten-containing products but also with most of the other carbs, including the gluten-free ones.

So he decided to open an antipasti bar and call it "Vivi's Antipasti Bar."

I loved this end so much that even when I decided to write the parable instead of the romance, I wanted to keep this scene in the book. Luca then became a secondary character, instead of the main one.

This happy ending elicited approving gasps and sighs from my fellow writers in our local writers' club. But even that reaction hadn't motivated me enough to continue working on either the parable or the romance.

Neither went much further than an unfinished plot-line and sketches of a few scenes.

Was it a failure on my part?

I don't think so now. After having written this "almost" memoir, I feel like the hero of my own parable, who has met and learned from so many amazing mentors. These mentors are my family, friends, doctors, nutrition and physiotherapy specialists, authors, fellow "intolerants" and "joint-achers," and many others. They are also the designers and players of their lives' games, and they design and play them in their own ways. I can learn so much by "looking over their shoulders." And then I can do what the legendary Bruce Lee famously suggested. I can "adapt what is useful, reject what is useless, and add what is specifically [my] own."

Below are the key lessons I have learned so far in my parable, while turning my life and the healing processes I choose and live through into fun games. I chose not to list them as bullet points, but instead write them down as paragraphs of flowing text as they come to me in waves of recognition and awareness. A list form feels like singular drops of a starting rain or jumping from one stepping stone to another while crossing a river. Let's follow the flow instead and start with the biggest wave.

Life is too precious and too short to be too serious about it. Smiles, the genuine ones that I feel not only on my face but also in my whole body, including my gut, are not serious. They are playful and gameful.

To turn my life into games, I need to be and do three things, or in other words, practice three skill sets: first, be here, then move one small step at a time, and finally, be and do both in a light, fun, and gameful way.

So if I am here truly with my mind and body instead of judging what I see and experience, and instead study it with curiosity and engagement as anthropologists do, then I can identify both the next, smallest and effortless step to take, and the most fun and exciting way to take and appreciate it.

No, I don't always manage to turn my life into fun games.

There is an occasional pity party when I eat what I am not supposed to or either skip a wellness exercise or do too much physically in one go and cause myself pain.

Sometimes I forget to be here and start considering what I have not good enough, and comparing what I can and cannot do with others. That leads to even greater pity parties, alright. But they are fortunately not as wild and dramatic as before.

Gluten is relatively easy to avoid because of how sick I get, and the occasional accidental contamination reminds me of this. Luckily this happens much less often than before.

Occasional pity parties result in me eating some milk products, chocolate, berries, fruits, or nuts. Shortly before Christmas 2019, I had some chocolate with nuts on several days in a row, and a half glass of white wine on a few of those days. What for others would go unnoticed resulted in a voice you'd get after a drunken party (not that I've had many of those in my life), a heavy and inflamed stomach, a bloated gut making me look several months pregnant (or a beer belly, as a friend once pointed out), constipation that made the bloating harder to cope with, restless nights waking up drenched in unpleasantly smelling sweat and needing increasingly frequent trips to the bathroom, more cramps in my feet and legs, and difficulty breathing through my nose. And to add to all that, my teeth and gums again became sensitive (sometimes with sores) to changes of temperature and hot or cold drinks.

I continue to learn that judging myself for these indulgences doesn't help me or the situation I am in. Being kind, honest, and caring while being fully here where I am with my mind and body, does.

I was inspired when I found a definition of the word 'health' by the acclaimed and super-prolific author Kristine Kathryn Rusch in her brilliant book *Writing with Chronic Illness*. Here it is:

"When I talk about health, I am talking about *self-care,* in all of its permutations."

So, in the spirit of taking good care of myself, I try to allow myself some indulgences without irritating my system. These indulgences don't have to be something sweet, in terms of confectionery. It can be an activity I am passionate about, such as writing or reading, or something that feels sweet and rejuvenating, be it spending time with my husband, playing a game with my children, or meeting with friends, in person or online. All I need to do is to test various options.

Looking at it all as an experiment feels like playing with those chemistry, physics, and weather-making sets for children.

If I look at it in a gameful and playful way, my life becomes such an exciting discovery set with endless opportunities to learn something new. Just like in the best game ever that has an endless number of levels to reach, but when you reach one, you feel like an all-time winner.

The same applies to all the other challenges that could be seen as fun challenges, including my eye condition and osteoarthritis. I can experiment with various types of exercises and movements and see what's fun for me and what doesn't irritate my body. Recently, I had this idea to do an eye exercise while also doing squats. So I took a little colorful crystal, held it in my hand, and brought it closer or farther away from my eyes while at the same time bending my knees and holding it for a few seconds. I had a lot of fun with this "double" exercise and experimenting with its different variants.

[A side-note added during the revision of this book: I have changed my "Well-Being" game design again. I separated eye gymnastics from body exercises once again. Who knows, I might find a way to bring them together once or many more times again. Here lies the brilliance of turning one's life into games. I don't ever have to stop playing with the designs of these games.]

I also discovered that I could look forward to the "games" suggested by others and try them out with an open and curious mind. That is how I feel about the physiotherapy for my left shoulder that my physician has referred me to. And I am hugely curious about the eye-test I have at the hospital in a couple of months.

Experimenting with how I record my awards (points, stars, donuts, and various types of badges) is enormous fun too. I change the colors, the names or number of the areas of my life I want to turn into games. Right now, I have three of these areas defined in the weekly calendar I call "Points, Stars, and Badges Gamebook." They are: "Creativity and Gratitude," "Well-Being," and "Sleep."

Everything I need to do for work, family, or home is "Creativity and Gratitude," and there are certain projects and activities I decide will get stars when worked on. I call this area of my life, which is connected to what I want and need to do (excepting those that contribute directly to my well-being, as below), "Creativity" because I can be creative in whatever I am up to. It was also its name before I added "Gratitude" to the title. I added "Gratitude" because at the end of the day, or during the day, I choose five areas I've been active in, of which I am particularly proud, and which deserve a star.

Along with this game, I sometimes play the "Appreciation Game," which is just a page in my project book (notebook) where I record each little step I accomplish during the day. That way, I make sure that I move in small steps and not in big jumps. After writing down what I just did, I immediately cross it out. For me, it closes the move, and I can then go to the next one.

This game is of big help on those days when my joints hurt most, my metabolism is off balance, or I am simply feeling down. All these recordings help me to become aware of everything I manage from day to day, from which I can choose some to win a star. Right now, I award five stars for five different activities I'm glad I did on that day. So you could say that I play a "Creative Game of Gratitude and Appreciation."

"Well-Being" ("the state of being comfortable, healthy, or happy" — Lexico[69]) is another "game" I play. It embraces various exercises for my eyes and body, as well as a place for a star if I don't consume any added sugar, fruits, nuts, or sugar alcohols (such as in wine, for example). And "Sleep" stands for getting enough sleep at night and from occasional daytime naps, where I get a star for at least seven hours in total. Lately, I have been experimenting with recording the nap time only if I had it before three in the afternoon. I read about this

---

[69] https://www.lexico.com/en/definition/well-being

recommendation on Bill Gates' blog[70]. So I am incorporating best practices and "testing" them for myself in my Self-Motivational Game Designs.

[An update: I recently merged the "Well-Being" and "Sleep" areas into one "Well-Being" area. You would agree that enough sleep contributes to our well-being. So, this move was natural. The rewards I get when I do something for my well-being are donuts. I draw and color them; each day gets a different color. Thus, the "Creativity and Gratitude" games bring me stars of appreciation (for myself by myself), and in the "Well-Being" games, I get donuts. For now, I collect (recorded here in alphabetical order) "Bouncing Donuts," "Eye Gymnastics Donuts," "No Sugar Donuts," "Sitting and Standing Donuts," "Sleeping Donuts," "Straight Posture Donuts," and "Walking Donuts." I'm curious about what other well-being games I will come up with in the future and what other quirky names for my rewards come out of that.]

Sometimes, the experiment can go "wrong," and my body's alarms go off. Or in other words, I lose the game, or I perceive it as having been lost. In truth, I never lose. Even my upsets are part of my daily games. In many games, like Tetris, losing is a major part of the design, and they are still loved by many. The players of these

---

[70] https://www.gatesnotes.com/Books/Why-We-Sleep?WT.mc_id=20191216012700_EOYBooks2019_BG-LI&WT.tsrc=BGLI&linkId=79019278

games don't feel like losers. They notice the number of points they gathered and try again.

I can view my daily experiences with my conditions the same way. I don't lose when I don't level up. My body's reactions are part of the game called life.

All I have to do when I "fail" is recover and repeat the experiment with adjusted parameters. Or, in game terms, you might say start the game again and try different moves than before to achieve the level. Or even re-design and then play it again.

Through all these experiences, I have learned that to live a happy life doesn't mean to live a constantly blissful life. That is impossible, and would be utterly dull if it was. To live a happy life is to experience ups and downs, like on a fun roller coaster. There, we don't feel like our lives are at stake or out of control, even if we don't know what the next curve will be like. We appreciate the surprising and sharp turns on a roller coaster. And the same is true of games. We appreciate the challenges games pose because we learn something new with each one.

We often perceive real-life situations as burdens, rather than something fun and exciting. We put too much drama on them instead of being open to experience them and discover something new.

A gameful life can lighten and brighten the real-life occurrences and help us to see them as a collection of brilliant games.

Yes, my life is a collection of many fun games. Each day is such an exciting collection.

Another beautiful thing happened along the way. I learned to trust my body. Trust that the experiences I have had so far are valid. Trust my body, my sanity. Trust myself. I forget that sometimes, but I recall it more often than before. That was one of the most important lessons on this journey.

My body does communicate with me a lot, including the bodily sensations of cold and heat and so on. Also, the possibly crazy thoughts my brain generates are signals that I (or my brain) need to interpret.

I am aware now of my delusion when I believed if I only overcame one challenge, I would never have another again. Now I see the colorful cocktail of my health conditions and challenges and remind myself that at any time another surprising ingredient might appear that I need to learn to incorporate so that the mixture works together. That might mean deliberately adding something of my own, like a new exercise or a new Self-Motivational Game, or the same ones with a new name and adjusted design.

I will also need to make sure I have a constant supply of fun, so my Fun Detecting Antenna needs to be around and switched on as long and as often as possible.

I hope I will never stop looking for analogies and parallels between what I have to deal with and anything gameful and playful. I imagine this hope inspired me to come up with the sweet and quirky character of Jen's grandmother in Vivi's story. I didn't have a name for her when I was plotting Vivi's story, but I had a clear idea of what kind of person she was. She loved video games and, even in her nineties, went to game conventions and competitions. Jen's grandmother lived her life as if it was a game and motivated Jen in my story to do the same.

That's what I hope for myself in my old age. And now as well. With that, I will serve not only myself and improve the quality of my life, but also the lives of others around me, especially my loved ones.

I am immensely happy and grateful to have seen and experienced many times that there are infinite ways to apply and test the tools (components) of Self-Gamification: awareness (anthropology), small steps (kaizen), and gamefulness (gamification).

Will I have more challenges to master, more levels to reach? Surely!

But it is up to me to make this process a fun game. The best thing about it is that I get all the freedom here, because:

I am both the designer and the player of the great collection of games called my life.

31. Now It's Your Turn

We all have things we struggle with or sides to ourselves that we resist and wish to be different.

Besides our fears, there are also physical challenges too.

More and more people have food intolerances and allergies. Or it could be something else entirely, with reactions or symptoms that aren't typical of either yourself or others.

But, you can learn not only to accept them, but to embrace them without judgment and even find sense in them, as well as learn how to treat yourself kindly, honestly, and helpfully.

Somewhere around the time I decided this book would be (mostly or at least partially) a memoir, I watched an interview that Sonia Sotomayor gave to Trevor Noah on the Daily Show, about her life as a Supreme Court Justice in the USA, her story with diabetes, and her new book for children *Just Ask!*[71].

Here is a quote from the book's description: "In *Just Ask*, United States Supreme Court Justice Sonia Sotomayor

---

[71] https://www.youtube.com/watch?v=Nztz3yuF3lY

celebrates the different abilities kids (and people of all ages) have"[72].

Her story with diabetes and the idea behind the book inspired me, so I immediately bought it for my children and also us parents. I have read the book many times with my children. It is beautiful and empowering. Yes, this book truly celebrates the different abilities of humans, which had been considered as disabilities in the past, but fortunately nowadays are seen as integral parts of humanity.

Here is one of my favorite bits in the book:

"Just like in our garden, all the ways we are different make our neighborhood — our whole world really — more interesting and fun. And just like all of these plants, each of us has unique powers to share with the world and make it more interesting and richer." — Sonia Sotomayor, *Just Ask!*

After watching Sonia Sotomayor's interview with Trevor Noah, and reading the book, I realized that we all need to share our experiences with others, regardless of whether they are going through the same thing or not.

So if, like me, you have certain challenges, especially if these are not visible to others, and they only become

---

[72] https://www.penguinrandomhouse.com/books/562056/just-ask-by-sonia-sotomayor-illustrated-by-rafael-lopez/

apparent in specific situations, then share your story with people. You never know how you might inspire others.

Practicing talking about your challenges will assist you in asking for help, which is critical in mastering them. Today I realized that when I tell people about my challenges and how I cope with them, I am sometimes indirectly asking for help. Then sometimes, in the middle of the telling, the listener has a great idea. Or I might even get the courage to ask directly for advice and help.

I fully understand that such sharing might be scary. Who knows what we might get in response, right? It might be a rejection, or some "crazy" or misplaced advice that we might feel obliged to follow. But if you observe yourself, the world around you, and your thought processes non-judgmentally, as well as permit yourself to process the information you get one little step at a time, and take on everything without losing your sense of humor, you will be able to maintain both kindness, honesty, and helpfulness toward yourself and those around you.

Here is a great tool to help you embrace the advice and information that others give you while trying to help, and enable you to appreciate their help full-heartedly, without deviating from your truth. It has helped me so many times, and Ariel and Shya Kane call this tool "True Listening." Here is what they say:

"True Listening is actively listening to another with the intention of hearing what is being said from the other's point of view."

And also,

"This act of listening is enough to pull you into the moment. However, you have an incredibly facile mind. You can race ahead in your thoughts and finish another person's sentence before he or she gets to the point. Or you can take exception to a word he or she uses and stop listening altogether. If you pay attention, you will see that there are many times when you have an internal commentary on what is being said rather than just listening. If you can train yourself to hear what is being said, from the speaker's point of view, it takes you outside of time and into the current moment." — Ariel and Shya Kane, *Working on Yourself Doesn't Work*

Thus, truly listen, without judgment. You might discover something entirely new and fresh, even in the things that have been said to you before.

You don't need to apply everything others advise you to do. It is your life and your health. Your game. Follow the advice of the legendary Bruce Lee, which I quoted in the previous chapter, but which is worth repeating:

"Adapt what is useful, reject what is useless, and add what is specifically your own."

Thus, trust your gut and "inner vision." If a suggestion comes and looms in your head (possibly through resistance to the advice given), but curiosity draws you to it over and over again, wondering how it would be to give it a try, then go ahead and give it a try. One, two, five, or more minutes at a time or on any particular day, but do it.

Don't forget to listen to your body. To yourself, really. Our bodies, including all their parts (also our brains), are amazing and give us so much information about our well-being. All we need to do is to truly listen and say, "Yes, I hear and appreciate you," without second-guessing and interpreting those signals.

And one more tip for your journey. If you feel an urge to share it with your family, friends, or on social media, do it. Kindly and honestly toward yourself and those with whom you share this information.

Here is another fantastic quote to encourage you to do so:

"Each person's 'ordinary' is another's 'extraordinary.' Being one's self and sharing that with others is simply a gift." — Ariel and Shya Kane, *Practical Enlightenment*

If this book touched you and as I hope helped you, then I invite you to share it with others, as well as the books I quoted and mention later in "Further Reading." Especially if they might be struggling with similar physical challenges to those described. Or maybe their loved ones would benefit from understanding what their child, parent, sibling, or partner is going through. All of them could profit from approaching health conditions gamefully.

Share with them the possibility of discovering their powers and ability to be the designer *and* the player of their lives, whatever their circumstances and state of mind.

 And last but not least, I invite you to share your stories with me, either on social media (you will find them on my website) or by e-mailing vib@optimistwriter.com.

I'd like to finish by posing the same question Sonia Sotomayor does in her book, just after the quote above,

"What will you do with your powers?" — Sonia Sotomayor, *Just Ask!*

Further Reading

In the chapter titled "3. Learning," I addressed what I have learned from books (among other things), and referred to them as my favorite teachers. Here are some of the books I learn from and how they help me.

Note: All lists are in alphabetical order.

To sharpen my skills in awareness and living in the moment, I will continue reading all the amazing books by Ariel and Shya Kane:

- *Being Here: Modern Day Tales of Enlightenment*, Ariel and Shya Kane, 2007

- *Being Here...Too: Short Stories of Modern Day Enlightenment*, Ariel and Shya Kane, 2018

- *How to Create a Magical Relationship: The 3 Simple Ideas that Will Instantaneously Transform Your Love Life*, Ariel and Shya Kane, 2008

- *How to Have A Match Made in Heaven: A Transformational Approach to Dating, Relating, and Marriage*, Ariel and Shya Kane, 2012

- *Practical Enlightenment*, Ariel and Shya Kane, 2015

- *Working on Yourself Doesn't Work: The 3 Simple Ideas That Will Instantaneously Transform Your Life*, Ariel and Shya Kane, 2008

When I want to recall how to make progress in small steps and to bypass my fears, I will call for help from:

- *One Small Step Can Change Your Life: The Kaizen Way*, Robert Maurer, 2014

- *Mastering Fear: Harnessing Emotion to Achieve Excellence in Work, Health and Relationships*, Robert Maurer, 2016

- *The Spirit of Kaizen: Creating Lasting Excellence One Small Step at a Time*, Robert Maurer, 2012

To learn from others who turn their health challenges into games, I will open and read:

- *SuperBetter: The Power of Living Gamefully*, Jane McGonigal, 2015

To embrace pain instead of resisting and fighting it, and to cope with challenges invisible to others, I am learning from:

- *How to Live Well with Chronic Pain and Illness: A Mindful Guide*, Toni Bernhard, 2015

To apply gentle pain relief techniques, I will learn, among others from:

- *Yoga for Pain Relief: Simple Practices to Calm Your Mind and Heal Your Chronic Pain*, Kelly McGonigal, 2009

To become aware of how to fuel and benefit my body and health in the best possible way, I will consult:

- *Eat Move Sleep: How Small Choices Lead to Big Changes*, Tom Rath, 2013

- *The Perfect Metabolism Plan*, by Sara Vance, 2015

To learn that I am not alone, how to include the differences of others, and how to feel included, for children and adults:

- *Just Ask! Be Different, Be Brave, Be You*, Sonia Sotomayor, Illustrated by Rafael López, 2019

To get me started when something appears daunting, I will find inspiration by reading the many great stories of everyday courage in:

- *The 5 Second Rule: Transform Your Life, Work, and Confidence with Everyday Courage*, Mel Robbins, 2017

Since this book is mostly a memoir, here is the book I chose to learn from, as I wrote it:

- *Fast-Draft Your Memoir: Write Your Life Story in 45 Hours*, Rachael Herron, 2018

Here are some of the memoirs I enjoy reading:

- *Dreams from My Father: A Story of Race and Inheritance*, Barack Obama, 2004

- *Eat, Pray, Love: One Woman's Search for Everything*, Elizabeth Gilbert, 2006

- *I'm Feeling Lucky: The Confessions of Google Employee Number 59*, Douglas Edwards, 2011

- *Maybe You Should Talk to Someone: A Therapist, HER Therapist, and Our Lives Revealed*, Lori Gottlieb, 2019

- *My Life as an Experiment: One Man's Humble Quest to Improve Himself by Living as a Woman, Becoming George*

Washington, Telling No Lies, and Other Radical Tests, A. J. Jacobs, 2010

- *Playing the Moldovans at Tennis*, Tony Hawks, 2013 (as well as his other memoirs)

- *Surely You're Joking Mr. Feynman! Adventures of a Curious Character*, Richard P. Feynman, 1985

Here are the parables that inspire me and which ignited a wish to write the parables in the "Gameful Life" series:

- *The Go-Giver: A Little Story About a Powerful Business Idea*, Bob Burg and John David Mann, 2010

- *The Go-Giver Influencer: A Little Story About a Most Persuasive Idea*, Bob Burg and John David Mann, 2018

- *The Go-Giver Leader: A Little Story About What Matters Most in Business*, Bob Burg and John David Mann, 2016

- *The Latte Factor: Why You Don't Have to Be Rich to Live Rich*, David Bach and John David Mann, 2019

- *The Recipe: A Story of Loss, Love, and the Ingredients of Greatness*, Charles M. Carroll and John David Mann, 2017

To continue being inspired as a writer, I currently consult several great writers on the writing craft, and how to be a professional writer whatever the circumstances:

- *The Healthy Writer: Reduce Your Pain, Improve Your Health, and Build a Writing Career for the Long Term*, Joanna Penn, 2017

- *The Mental Game of Writing: How to Overcome Obstacles, Stay Creative and Productive, and Free Your Mind for Success*, James Scott Bell, 2016

- *Writing with Chronic Illness: Improve Outlook and Productivity*, Kristine Kathryn Rusch, 2019

Acknowledgments

I am a lucky person to be blessed with such an abundance of kind people in my life. It would take more than a book to thank everyone who has affected my life and this book. So, instead of thanking each person individually, I will thank groups of people. Only a handful of people will be mentioned by name here. And you will see why below.

First of all, dear reader, thank you very much for purchasing and reading *Gameful Healing*!

My favorite teachers are books, and I will always be grateful to the many talented and inspiring people creating these beautiful wells of wisdom, inspiration, and encouragement.

I would like to thank all of the doctors, nurses, and health specialists who provided medical care, advice, and help when I both needed and asked for it, and when I was sometimes afraid to ask for it.

Big and heartfelt thanks to all fellow "intolerants," "thalassemia bearers," "Bell's-palsiers," and "joint-achers." Thank you for sharing your experiences with me, either in person or through your magazines, blogs, and social media. A special shout out to the German and

Danish Celiac Associations. I learned a lot from being a member of both.

Huge thanks to my friends in the Black Label Writers Club in Aalborg for your honest and kind feedback on the early versions (novel and parable outlines) of this book.

My family, both on my husband's and my side, are all simply amazing at taking good care of me, and making salads when I come to visit. There are so many of you in all the branches of our big family, and each one of you is simply wonderful.

And here are the few callouts by name.

Dear Jen, thank you for your interest in this book, and suggestion to keep in touch and share our writing projects. Thank you also for your inspiring blog. It served as great research material.

Vang, thank you so, so much for the challenge with the bouncing, hopping, and breathing exercise. It had such an amazing impact on me. Dear Hien, thank you for suggesting a variant of jumping jacks (star jumps) to extend my hopping and bouncing workout. It added much fun and relaxed many muscles, especially in my shoulders.

I am hugely grateful to Alice Jago for editing this book. I enjoy reading my books after you have edited them. They sound so much better! Thank you so, so much!

My most heartfelt thanks go to my husband, Michael, and our children Niklas and Emma. This book wouldn't exist without you. I love you!

About the Author

Victoria is a writer, coach, and consultant with a background in semiconductor physics, electronic engineering (with a Ph.D.), information technology, and business development. While being a non-gamer, Victoria came up with the term Self-Gamification, a gameful and playful self-help approach bringing anthropology, kaizen, and gamification-based methods together to increase the quality of life. She approaches all areas of her life this way. Due to the fun she has turning everything in her life into games, she intends never to stop designing and playing them.

Victoria is the author of the *5 Minute Perseverance Game, Self-Gamification Happiness Formula, Gameful Project Management,* and *The Who, What, When, Where, Why & How of Turning Life into Fun Games* as well as the instructor of the online course, *Motivate Yourself by Turning Your Life Into Fun Games. Gameful Healing* is Victoria's sixth work (and the second book in the "Gameful Life" series) on how to approach projects, activities, health conditions, and life with excellence and ease in a gameful way — the Self-Gamification way.

Victoria was born in Moldova, lived in Germany for twelve years, and now lives in Aalborg, Denmark, with her husband and two children.

Visit or contact Victoria at

victoriaichizlibartels.com or optimistwriter.com.

Subscribe to Victoria's blog and news at

www.victoriaichizlibartels.com/subscribe-to-victorias-blog/.

To read about and join the Self-Gamification community go to

www.victoriaichizlibartels.com/community/.

By Victoria Ichizli-Bartels

Motivational Books

"Gameful Life" Series
Gameful Project Management:
Self-Gamification Based Awareness Booster for Your Project
Management Success
(Gameful Life Book 1)

Gameful Healing:
Almost a Memoir; Not Quite a Parable
(Gameful Life Book 2)
This book

Gameful Writing:
Seven People, Seven Stories, Seven Lessons Learned
(Gameful Life Book 3)
To be published in Spring/Summer 2020

Standalone Books
The Who, What, When, Where, Why & How of Turning Life into
Fun Games:
A Compressed Version of the Self-Gamification Happiness Formula

Self-Gamification Happiness Formula:
How to Turn Your Life into Fun Games

Gameful Healing

5 Minute Perseverance Game:
Play Daily for a Month and Become the Ultimate Procrastination Breaker

Cheerleading for Writers:
Discover How Truly Talented You Are

Turn Your No Into Yes:
15 Yes-Or-No Questions to Disentangle Your Project
Free e-book
(Available upon subscription to victoriaichizlibartels.com or optimistwriter.com)

Online Course
Motivate Yourself by Turning Your Life Into Fun Games:
Practice Self-Gamification, a Unique Self-Help Approach Uniting Anthropology, Kaizen, and Gamification
www.udemy.com/course/motivate-yourself-by-turning-your-life-into-fun-games/

Business
Books
Take Control of Your Business:
Learn what Business Rules are, discover that you are already using them, then update them to maximize your business success

Resources
The Business Rules Memo
www.victoriaichizlibartels.com/s1000d-navigation-maps/#BrMemo

S1000D
Books
brDoc, BREX, and Co.: S1000D Business Rules Made Easier

S1000D® Issue 4.1 and Issue 4.2 Navigation Map:
552+87 and 427+90 Business Rule Decision Points Arranged into two Linear Topic Maps to Facilitate Learning, Understanding, and Implementation of S1000D®

S1000D Issue 4.1 Untangled:
552+ Business Rules Decision Points Arranged into a Linear Topic Map to Facilitate Learning, Understanding and Implementation of S1000D
(unpublished, replaced by *S1000D® Issue 4.1 and Issue 4.2 Navigation Map,* see above)

Data Sheets and Templates
S1000D® Navigation Maps
www.victoriaichizlibartels.com/s1000d-navigation-maps/

Fiction
Books
Between Grace and Abyss: A Short Story
(Also available as a free e-book upon subscription to victoriaichizlibartels.com or optimistwriter.com)

Nothing Is As It Seems: A Novelette
(The e-book is permanently free)

Gameful Healing

Seven Broken Pieces: A short story
(Prequel to series "A Life Upside Down")

A Spy's Daughter: A novella
(Book 1 in series "A Life Upside Down")

The Truth About Family:
A novel inspired by true events